Asperger Syndrome

A Guide for Professionals and Families

Issues in Children's and Families' Lives

Series Editors:
Thomas P. Gullotta, *Child and Family Agency of Southeastern Connecticut, New London, Connecticut*
Herbert J. Walberg, *University of Illinois at Chicago, Chicago, Illinois*
Roger P. Weissberg, *University of Illinois at Chicago, Chicago, Illinois*

ASPERGER SYNDROME
A Guide for Professionals and Families
Edited by Raymond W. DuCharme and Thomas P. Gullotta

CHANGING WELFARE
Edited by Rachel A. Gordon and Herbert J. Walberg

PREVENTING YOUTH PROBLEMS
Edited by Anthony Biglan, Margaret C. Wang, and Herbert J. Walberg

A Continuation Order Plan is available for this series. A continuation order will bring delivery of each new volume immediately upon publication. Volumes are billed only upon actual shipment. For further information please contact the publisher.

Asperger Syndrome
A Guide for Professionals and Families

Edited by

Raymond W. DuCharme

The Learning Clinic, Inc.
Brooklyn, Connecticut

and

Thomas P. Gullotta

Child and Family Agency of Southeastern Connecticut
New London, Connecticut

Research Assistants

Jessica M. Ramos
Child and Family Agency of Southeastern Connecticut
New London, Connecticut

and

Jennifer C. Messina
Villanova University Villanova, Pennsylvania

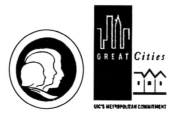

GREAT *Cities*

UIC'S METROPOLITAN COMMITMENT

Kluwer Academic / Plenum Publishers
New York • Boston • Dordrecht • London • Moscow

Library of Congress Cataloging-in-Publication Data

Asperger syndrome : a guide for professionals and families / edited by Raymond
   W. DuCharme and Thomas P. Gullotta.
      p.   cm.—(Issues in children's and families' lives)
   Includes bibliographical references and index.
   ISBN 0-306-47867-6
   1. Asperger's syndrome.   2. Asperger's syndrome—Patients—Family relationships.
   3. Parents of autistic children.   I. DuCharme, Raymond W.   II. Gullotta, Thomas,
   1948–   III. Series.

RJ506.A9A855   2004
362.198′928588—dc22   2003054469

ISBN: 0-306-47867-6

© 2003 by Kluwer Academic/Plenum Publishers
233 Spring Street, New York, New York 10013

http://www.wkap.nl/

10 9 8 7 6 5 4 3 2 1

A C.I.P. record for this book is available from the Library of Congress

Permission for books published in Europe: permissions@wkap.nl
Permissions for books published in the United States of America: permissions@wkap.com

Printed in the United States of America

To R.S. and R.B. for both of whom I need to have better answers
R.W.D.

Preface

Every book has not one but many stories to tell as readers bring their life experience and unique personal interpretation to the words found on those written pages. For Tom Gullotta, this book began unknowingly some nineteen or so years ago with the adoption of his three-week-old son. Bernie's inexhaustible energy, excitability, and precocious self-centered nature had created by kindergarten a record already inches thick. To this history still more feet of documentation, conflicting opinions, and, frankly, anguish would be added before the words Asperger Syndrome (AS) were first mentioned at age fourteen. Tom suspects that many readers with children or other loved ones with AS have had similar experiences.

For Raymond DuCharme, this book is part of a long search for ways to help children and their families. He states,

> Children teach us a great deal about ourselves, and fragile children teach us to be thoughtful about our effects on them. A child's reaction mirrors our sensitivity, or our lack of sensitivity.
>
> Children with AS are among the most fragile children. They are most reactive to what they are not prepared to do. They have taught me that I must use their signals to adjust my expectations, and to tap their potential. They have taught me to use the evidence that they provide to help them do what they most wish—to be as accepted and as successful as their peers.

From these different journeys, this volume was conceived as a Hartman Scholar's program. Nearly a decade since its inception, Hartman Scholar programs identify an issue affecting children and their families for intensive study. Once an issue has been selected for study, a search is undertaken to identify leading scholars and practitioners working in that area. To be a Hartman Scholar is demanding, entailing two weekend study groups over a period of one year, with individual study occurring between meetings. The product of that year-long collaboration is the volume before you.

The eight chapters that follow cluster into three untitled sections. The first, consisting of four chapters, provides readers with a comprehensive overview of the syndrome. In Chapter 1, Raymond DuCharme and Kathleen McGrady examine the etiology of AS and address the confusion that surrounds diagnostic issues pertaining to it. In Chapter 2, Brenda Myles examines the evidence-based literature and identifies programs that show promise. In Chapter 3, Raymond DuCharme provides a comprehensive overview of instructional studies. This review is enriched with a wealth of additional data from the author's work at The Learning Clinic, which points to an educational approach that is successful with youth with AS. In Chapter 4, the first section concludes with an examination by Ann Wagner and Kathleen McGrady of counseling and other therapeutic strategies that are helpful to youth with AS and their families.

The second grouping of chapters focuses on two critical issues affecting youth with AS. Chapter 5 by Liza Little examines the risk these young people face for victimization and strategies toward reducing that risk. In Chapter 6, Peter F. Gerhardt explores the subject of transition support for learners with AS from childhood into adulthood. He identifies several areas in which substantial work remains to be undertaken if the lives of these deserving individuals are to be maximized.

The final grouping of chapters are of special importance. Chapter 7 by Sherry Moyer and Sheryl Breetz offers not only practical advice from the mother of a young person with AS but also provides a case study in how transitional housing and support services can be developed for young people as they "age out" of the educational system. Chapter 8 by Stephen Shore is a positive, hopeful, often times humorous accounting of Stephen's life with AS. In a conversational tone that connects with the experiences of individuals with AS and their families, this remarkable young man helps all of us to understand AS much better.

We offer this book to policymakers, educators, practitioners, and graduate students, but most of all to individuals with AS and the families of individuals with AS. We hope that policymakers will use the lessons found in this volume to craft laws and funding opportunities that serve this underserved and often unrecognized population. We hope that educators and practitioners apply the scant knowledge that is available and join us in calling for intensified efforts to develop evidence-based services for individuals with AS. We hope that this work serves as a motivational starting point for students to undertake badly needed research to improve the dearth of knowledge in this area. But most of all, we offer this book to the Bernies who live with AS every day of their lives and to their parents who love them so dearly. May this book not only offer some hope but inspire you to speak out on behalf of all with AS.

RAYMOND W. DUCHARME
THOMAS P. GULLOTTA

Acknowledgments

A project of this scope and magnitude requires support and assistance at many different levels. Tom Gullotta is indebted to John and Kelly Hartman for enabling this program to be established. He expresses his deepest appreciation to the Board of Child and Family Agency of Southeastern Connecticut who have encouraged him over many years to actively pursue knowledge and to turn that knowledge with other staff into practices that enable families to succeed. Further, this effort would have not been successful were it not for assistance from the Connecticut Department of Mental Health and Addiction Services. In particular, thanks goes to Commissioner Thomas Kirk and to Dianne Harnad, Director of Prevention Services. Research assistants Jessica Ramos and Jennifer Messina provided valuable copyediting, proofreading, and library research support for which Tom and Ray are grateful. At Child and Family, the logistic responsibilities for this program fell on the very able shoulders of Judy Lovelace, whose charm, grace, and competence ensures that this effort runs smoothly. Raymond DuCharme reflects back on the start of his career and acknowledges the lasting influence on him by Delores Taylor, Ph.D. and Jim Simmons, M.D. for their simple, clear advice and guidance. Both are dedicated to the value of research and the need to apply it to meet the needs of children and their families.

Contents

Asperger Syndrome

A Guide for Professionals and Families

Chapter 1

What Is Asperger Syndrome?

Raymond W. DuCharme and Kathleen A. McGrady

Review of the Literature

Over the last decade, researchers have explored the basis for Asperger Syndrome. Some of that research yields evidence that resolves the question, Does Asperger Syndrome exist?

A search of the literature using the keyword "Asperger" produced three hundred eighty-five studies, articles, and other references. One hundred sixty-six studies pertained to diagnosis. The researchers whose purpose was to clarify issues related to the validity of Asperger Syndrome are the primary sources for the following discussion. Their articles examine the requirements of a system that differentiates among autism, Asperger Syndrome, High Functioning Autism, Pervasive Developmental Delay, Not Otherwise Specified and Non-Verbal Learning Disability.

Raja and Azzoni (2001) discuss the autistic condition described almost simultaneously by Dr. Asperger in Vienna (in 1944) and Dr. Kanner (in 1943) in Baltimore. Both men were medically trained in Vienna at about the same time.

Dr. Kanner (1943) described the characteristics of children that he diagnosed as having infantile autism. Dr. Asperger (1944) made observations of children in his hospital unit in Vienna that he characterized as "autistic psychopathy" (Frith, 1991). Dr. Kanner's diagnosis of infantile autism is more severe than Dr. Asperger's label. Their work has inspired decades of research that attempts to clarify the differences and similarities between the two clinical descriptions.

In recent years Asperger Syndrome (AS) was considered to be a pervasive developmental disorder (PDD) and was included as a new diagnosis in the *World Health Organization International Classification of Diseases* (ICD-10) (1992) and the United States (1994) *Diagnostic and Statistical Manual of Mental Disorders,* Fourth Edition (DSM-IV) (APA, 1994). For a comparison of factors included in the diagnoses, see the table below.

Asperger Syndrome Criteria

	DSM-IV	ICD-10
Qualitative impairment in social interaction	X	X
Restricted, repetitive, and stereotyped patterns of behavior, interests, and activities	X	X
No general language delay	X	X
No delay in cognitive development	X	X
Normal general intelligence (most)		X
Markedly clumsy (common)		X
No delay in development of:		
age-appropriate self-help skills		
adaptive behavior (excluding social interaction)	X	
curiosity about environment		

Eisenmajer et al. (1996) point out that the DSM-IV criteria for Asperger's Disorder (AsD), (now called Asperger Syndrome), is the same as that for Autism Disorder (AD) with three exceptions:

1. Communication and imagination impairment criteria for AD are not listed for ASD.
2. The child with an ASD diagnosis is described not to suffer from a clinically significant general delay in language; e.g. single words by age 2 years and phrases by age 3.
3. The child with ASD does not have a clinically significant delay in cognitive development or in the development of age appropriate self-help skills, adaptive behavior and curiosity about the environment.

Raja and Azzoni (2001) state that "the syndrome Hans Asperger originally described may not be captured by the present DSM-IV or ICD-10 criteria".

There are differences between the diagnostic criteria provided by the DSM-IV and the ICD-10. While the ICD-10 endorses the traits of normal intelligence and clumsy behavior, the DSM-IV does not include those traits. Further, the DSM-IV lists that there is no delay in the development of age appropriate self-help skills, adaptive behavior (excluding social interaction), and curiosity about the environment. Note that the ICD-10 does not list these criteria.

Behavior Patterns

Fundamental differences in criteria produce a serious threat to the external validity of the diagnosis of Asperger Syndrome. The similarity between an Autistic Disorder diagnosis and a Pervasive Developmental Disorder Not Otherwise Specified (PDD NOS) diagnosis adds to the difficulty in interpreting diagnostic categories.

Leekham et al. (2000) developed algorithms for a Diagnostic Interview for Social and Communication Disorders (DISCO). The interview models were used to compare the ICD-10 for AS with those developed by Gillberg in 1993. Two hundred (200) children and adults were studied, all of whom met the ICD-10 criteria for childhood autism or atypical autism. Only 1% met the ICD-10 criteria for AS. Forty-five (45) percent of the sample met the AS criteria defined by Gillberg. The study revealed that the discrepancy in diagnoses was due to the ICD-10 requirement for "normal" development of cognitive skills. Gillberg's criteria showed that the participants diagnosed with AS differed significantly from others on all but two Gillberg criteria. The authors question the benefit of defining a separate AS sub group. They suggest, as do Klin et al. (1995), Volkmar et al. (1998), and Schopler et al. (1998) that a dimensional view of the autistic spectrum is more appropriate than a categorical one. The definition of a "syndrome" or pattern of symptoms along a continuum is more useful than the term "disorder".

Gillberg's six criteria (Ehlers & Gillberg 1993) comprise social impairments, narrow interests, repetitive routines, speech and language peculiarities, non-verbal communication problems and motor clumsiness. Gillberg includes Szatmari et al. (1989) criteria and Tantam's (1988) five criteria. The ICD-10 and DSM-IV note an absence of any clinical delay in language and cognitive development in the first 3 years of life. The DSM-IV adds no delay in the development of self-help skills, adaptive behavior, and curiosity about the environment.

The broader criteria of Gillberg (1993), Szatmari et al. (1989), Tantam (1988) appear to differentiate between groups more reliably than do the DSM-IV and ICD-10. However, the interview structure of the DISCO requires that parents demonstrate an accurate description of symptoms and degree of severity. The DISCO algorithms do provide for decisions about the level of severity for item quantification.

It is also important to note that the developmental signpost of 3 years of age for evidence of delays may be too limiting, as critical functions may become deficient over time, through subsequent developmental stages. Also, the criterion of an IQ of 70 or above may place the lower level too low, given the normal range of IQ that other researchers use as the standard for an AS characteristic. Other research (DuCharme & McGrady, 2003) suggest that patterns of pragmatic skill deficits persist across ages for AS individuals. These language patterns require further investigation.

Measurement Tools

Screening tools are now available. Some examples are the (CAST) Childhood Asperger Syndrome Test (Scott, Baron-Cohen, Bolton, Brayne, 2002), The Asperger Syndrome Diagnostic Scale (Myles, Bock, & Simpson, 2001), Austim Spectrum Screening Questionnaire (ASSQ) (Ehlers, Gillberg, Wing, 1999) and the Gillberg DISCO model, Diagnostic Interview for Social and Communication Disorders (Leekham, Libby, Wing, Gould & Gillberg, 2000). The growing use of such measures is welcome. A recent article in *Exceptional Parent* (March 2003, pp. 104–107) revealed that very few children are provided with standardized developmental screening by their pediatricians. Early identification and intervention are not standard practice.

The Developmental Behavior Checklist is reported by Tonge et al. (1999) to identify behavioral and emotional disturbance present in the functioning of HFA and AS children and adolescents. The authors report patterns of disruptive, "anxious," autistic/social relating and anti-social behaviors to be measurable concomitants of Asperger Syndrome. In overall severity of psychopathology, the AS group scored significantly higher than the autism group. The differences were not due to age or intellectual level.

By administering a combination of the available assessment tools, educators now have the ability to identify problems in the areas of language and communication skills, level of social adjustment, indices of maladaptive behavior, cognitive functioning, and sensory motor development. The types and severity of maladaptive behavioral symptoms require further investigation to determine whether a dual diagnosis is indicated.

Comparing Diagnoses

Research suggests that a dimensional view of the autism spectrum is more appropriate than the categorical approach represented by the ICD-10 and DSM-IV. A dimensional view considers patterns of symptoms, or characteristics, and degrees of severity.

Ozonoff et al. (2000) compared twenty-three (23) children with HFA with twelve (12) children who were diagnosed with AS. Both groups were matched for chronological age, gender and intellectual ability. The sources of difference between the groups are categorized as cognitive functions, current symptoms, and early history. The authors conclude that HFA and AS involve the same symptomatology and differ only in degree of severity.

When comparing length of time in special education, the authors found that HFA students remained in special education self-contained classes longer than AS students.

Klin et al. (1995) report on the validity of neuropsychological characterization of Asperger Syndrome and the convergence of AS with Non-Verbal Learning Disability. Their research used the ICD-10 diagnostic criteria. The authors compared neuropsychological profiles of Asperger Syndrome (AS) and High Functioning Autism (HFA) and the assets and deficits described by the term "non-verbal learning disability" (NLD) reported by Rourke (1995). The groups were described to differ significantly in eleven neuropsychological areas.

The aspects of NLD, typical of child functioning, include deficits in tactile perception, psycho-motor coordination, visual-spatial organization, non-verbal problem solving, appreciation of incongruity, and humor. The NLD child demonstrates poor pragmatic language skill and impaired prosody in speech, along with deficits in social perception, social judgment and social interaction skills. All of these examples of child functioning for NLD are also typical of the AS child. Both groups, AS and NLD, also share the tendency toward social withdrawal and mood disorder (Klin et al. 1995, p. 1130). NLD is not part of the diagnostic nosology of either the ICD-10 or DSM-IV.

Schopler and Mesibov (1998) identify the similar characteristics of HFA and AS. They support the notion of "symptom overlap" between Autism, High-Functioning Autism, and Asperger Sydrome. Manjiviona and Prior (1999) reported that higher IQ scores among AS students account for differences. Klin et al. (1995) reported that although the AS and HFA groups did not differ in full scale IQ, the verbal – performance differential (VIQ – PIQ) were significantly different. The AS group demonstrated a higher verbal IQ and lower performance IQ in comparison to the HFA group.

The degree of overlap between the psychiatric diagnosis AS/HFA, and the neuropsychological characterization of NLD, indicates a high degree of concordance between AS and NLD. The neuropsychological description of assets and deficits (NLD) is a model for AS, but not for HFA. It is not useful then to identify Non-verbal Learning Disability as a separate diagnostic group apart from Asperger Syndrome.

Prevalence reports are limited by the validity measures associated with basic researches. The lack of agreement on diagnostic criteria may result in unreliable estimations. Lord, Rutter, & Le Couteur (1994) reported the prevalence of Autism to be 2–4 per 10,000 students. Wing (1993) reported one percent of the population and Gillberg (1995) 6.5 per 10,000 students. Ehlers and Gillberg (1993) report the prevalence of Asperger Syndrome to be 26–36 per 10,000 school age subjects.

Klin et al. (1995) conclude that AS appears to be a "very mild" form of PDD. The authors question the face value of creating the AS grouping apart form the PDD NOS category.

The validity of research findings is clearly dependent upon the clarity and reliability of the classification assigned to the subject. If a subject is wrongly classified as AS, or HFA, or PDD, any research based on that subject is flawed.

Characteristics of Asperger Syndrome

Motor Development

It is reported that delayed motor milestones and presence of motor clumsiness are AS characteristics. But there is a paucity of research to corroborate a clear association between motor delay and other AS characteristics (Ghaziuddin & Butler, 1998).

Motor delay and early language delay prior to age three are not predictive of other AS characteristics or of later developmental problems. The definition of "language delay" may be too limited as this usually pertains to the child's saying single word or simple phase.

Motor development and "clumsiness" were investigated by Ghaziuddin, and Butler (1998), Ghaziuddin et al. (1994). The authors found no significant relationship between coordination scores and diagnostic category after adjusting scores for intelligence.

Weimer et al. (2001) suggest that the motor clumsiness reported by Green et al. (2002) and Miyahara et al. (1997) may be the proprioceptive deficits that underlie the cases of uncoordination observed in some AS cases.

Speech and Prosody

Shriberg et al. (2001) investigated the speech and prosody characteristics of adolescents and adults with HFA and AS. Prosody includes phrasing, variability in speech production, same word duration in sentences, and grammatical placement of stressed and unstressed syllables and words. Voice loudness, pitch and quality were also compared.

Volubility differences and articulation errors, suggest minor differences between AS and HFA subjects. There was a high prevalence of speech-sound distortion in both groups. AS subjects used higher volume.

Findings associated with prosody and voice analyses identified significant differences between clinical and control groups in the areas of phrasing, stress, and nasal resonance. Two-thirds of the AS speakers were coded as having non-fluent phrasing on more than 20% of their utterances. It is speculated that repetition and revision may be related to formulation difficulties. There is also a suggestion that length of utterance is associated with phrasing errors. Higher levels of grammatical complexity were also associated with phrasing errors and length of utterance.

Gilchrist et al. (2001) compared adolescent AS, HFA, and Conduct Disorder (DO) diagnoses as to behavioral and speech abnormalities. The AS group demonstrated less severe behavioral abnormalities than the autism group and were unlikely to have speech abnormalities. The AS group had other communicative and social behavior difficulties similar to HFA. The AS group did better in structured one-to-one conversation than other groups.

Language and Meaning

Jolliffe and Baron-Cohen (2000) examined linguistic processing in high functioning adults with autism or AS. The ability to establish causal connections and to interrelate "local chunks" into higher-order "chunks" so that most linguistic elements are linked together thematically is defined as "global coherence". The authors hypothesized that adults on the Autism Spectrum, including AS, would have difficulty integrating information so as to derive meaning. Results showed that the clinical groups were less able to arrange sentences coherently and to use context to make a global inference.

The findings of the study on the abilities called "global coherence" are inconsistent with classroom experience with adolescent HFA and AS student performance at TLC (DuCharme & McGrady, 2003). Thirty (30) students were given a task with directions for writing a news story; seven statements of instruction; and ten individual descriptive informational statements, six of which are relevant to a theme, and four, irrelevant. The assignment was to create a news story that has a main point by selecting relevant information from the sentences provided. All thirty (30) students successfully completed the task, but demonstrated an inability to select information less relevant or irrelevant to the main theme.

Jolliffe and Baron-Cohen (2000) require an inference and use of connotative meaning to demonstrate comprehension. Global coherence may be different from inference. TLC student behavior demonstrated the ability to identify a main theme and related, supporting data that are "coherent." No inference was required.

The "global coherence" requirement of the Jolliffe & Baron-Cohen (2000) study to interpret and infer within the context of a story is different from combining facts into a coherent statement or conclusion. The definition of their task has connotative implications. Connotative and denotative meaning derive from linguistic processes that may differ from the processes used to infer meaning from factual content.

Frith (1991), Minshew et al. (1995) describe linguistic difficulties present when an AS person is given complex interpretive language tasks. Deficits are found in complex information processing abilities. However, linguistic basic skills are preserved.

Channon et al. (2001) presented video taped real-life problems to thirty (30) pre-teen and adolescent youth. Fifteen (15) were diagnosed AS and fifteen (15) were placed in a control group. The AS group differed in their ability to provide socially appropriate solutions to the problems as compared to the control group responses. The inability to draw inferences and to define appropriate attribution to key factors present in social situations are also discussed by Barnhill (2001) and Barnhill and Myles (2001).

Cognitive Processes

Cognitive flexibility required to solve a novel problem or a familiar problem in a novel situation is absent for AS persons to a degree beyond what their normal to superior IQ score should predict. Shulman et al. (1995) report that individuals on the Autism Spectrum have difficulties with tasks that necessitate internal manipulation of information.

Theory of Mind (TOM) is defined as the ability to infer mental states, including beliefs, intentions and thoughts (Perner & Wimmer, 1985). Happe (1995) describes these internalized manipulations of information as mentalizing. How "mentalizing" is related to "global coherence" and TOM is unclear. But these processes suggest an interface among auditory processing, language, cognition, and the "load" of factors present in any situation.

Dunn et al. (2002) support, with preliminary evidence, the view that clear differences exist in the sensory processing patterns of children with AS when compared with non-clinical peers. AS students are reported to have difficulty with auditory processing; they demonstrate poor ability to modulate their responses from one situation to another. The authors advocate for a student to receive a sensory measurement that will yield a profile that reflects the assessment of sensory processing, modulation of behavioral-emotional responses and level of response to "sensory events." Sensory processing deficits may alter the ability to cognitively manipulate data accurately.

The observations by Frith (1991) and Frith and Happe (1994) that AS children are limited in their ability to demonstrate pretend play, imagination and creativity has some support in the research literature (Craig and Baron-Cohen, 1999). This apparent restricted ability to predict future events by manipulating past experience, as part of problem solving, may be related to measures of limited creativity and TOM factors identified early in AS child development (Baron-Cohen et al., 1999) (Jolliffe & Baron-Cohen, 2000).

Ehlers et al. (1997) compared the cognitive profiles of AS, AD, and ADD students 5 to 15 years old. The Swedish version of WISC III, the Kaufman Factors of Verbal Comprehension, Perceptual Organization and Freedom from Distractibility measurements were compared for forty (40) students in each group. The AS and AD groups differed in respect to "fluid" and "crystallized" cognitive ability. The Kaufman Factor scores accounted for more variance than WISC III Verbal or Performance IQ scores.

De Leon et al. (1986), Courchesne et al. (1994), Schultz et al. (2000), Morris et al. (1999) investigated brain hemisphere function associated with developmental prosopagnosia and visual-perceptual functions involved in face recognition. There is inconclusive evidence that inability to perceive emotion in facial cues is a neurocognitive dysfunction of visual-perception (Grossman et al. 2000). The conclusion does not imply that there is no evidence of cortical neuropathology present in Asperger Syndrome. Casanova et al. (2002), Rourke et al. (1983), Aman et al. (1998).

Asperger Syndrome Profile

Barnhill (2001) provides a synthesis of research conducted by the "AS Project". The AS Project was designed to provide an "empirically valid profile of individuals with AS" p. 300. A series of studies is summarized to provide a description of AS children and youth. The following characteristics are reported:

1. IQs similar to the general population, ranging from deficient to very superior.
2. Significantly less capable written than oral language skills.
3. Limited ability to problem solve in contrast to verbal fluency skill.

4. Measured emotional difficulties not endorsed by the AS students themselves.
5. Problems with inferential comprehension.
6. Attributions that parallel a learned helplessness approach.
7. Sensory problems similar to a cognitively deficient person.

It is helpful to separate the influence of intelligence quotient from each diagnostic classification; e.g. autism IQ quotient in the deficient range and AS IQ quotient in the normal to very superior range. Barnhill (2000) omits other characteristics such as eye gaze, pragmatic language deficiencies, poor speech characteristics of prosody, volume, phrasing, grammatical structure and word stress.

The cluster of factors associated with socialization, social skill development and social reality testing are important discriminant variables associated with Asperger Syndrome. The tendency to prefer aloneness, to avoid peers in preference to adult interaction, other avoidant behaviors, and marginal independent living skills are also related to diagnosis and prognosis for AS persons (Nesbitt, 2000) (Matthews, 1996) (Mawhood & Howlin, 1999) ((Tantam, 2000) (Dewey, 1991) (Dyer et al., 1996).

The inability to draw inferences, to interpret connotative meaning, and to apprehend relationships between factual knowledge and higher order thinking also need to be included as AS characteristics worthy of investigation. Evidence of over and under reactivity to ordinary stimuli, and attentional shift problems are important characteristics (Courchesne et al., 1994). Level of cognitive rigidity in the presence of anxiety producing stimuli reported anecdotally has important heurestic value in future researches.

AS is a complex continuum of symptoms that are suggested by the various researchers and these problematic symptoms of communication and language, cognition, adaptability, lack of generalization of skill, socialization and sensory processing are more evident in the interactions that are part of the daily activities of natural environment than the testing room. The clarity of the diagnostic nosology is important. And the need to assess AS persons as part of the natural daily routine is also important in order to obtain a valid assessment of competencies.

Associated Co-morbid Conditions

The effort to obtain an accurate diagnosis and treatment for an Asperger child is usually not straight forward. AS is a multi-faceted disorder with subtle manifestation of deficits (Mesibov et al., 2001). The diagnostic process is further complicated by co-morbid conditions, or other secondary problematic behaviors. These may include difficulties with attention and concentration, anxious behaviors, depression, motor or vocal tics, obsessive-compulsive behaviors, noncompliant or aggressive behaviors, or learning disabilities (Klin, Volkmar & Sparrow, 2000). Behaviors associated with these conditions tend to be disruptive, and therefore become the focus of treatment and diagnosis. Before it is recognized that a youngster has AS, the child may be given one or more of the following diagnostic labels: Attention-Deficit/Hyperactivity Disorder (ADHD), Depression, Anxiety Disorder, Obsessive Compulsive Disorder (OCD), Oppositional-Defiant Disorder, or Schizophrenia. In some cases the child may have a co-morbid condition, which warrants the diagnosis. In other cases, the behaviors are a manifestation of one of the many features of AS, and do not meet the criteria for a second diagnosis.

Attention-Deficit/Hyperactivity Disorder

Difficulties with attention and concentration are not uncommon with AS children, especially in younger children (Klin, Volkmar, & Sparrow, 2000). According to Klin and Volkmar (1997) 28% of AS children have a comorbid diagnosis of ADHD. However, the AS child can present with impaired attention without having ADHD. Some features of AS that interfere with attention include sensory overload, and fixated attention. With sensory overload, the AS child has difficulty filtering out irrelevant stimuli, and can become overloaded with sensory input. Instead of focusing attention on what is relevant, he or she is "distracted" by too much sensory input, failing to attend to what is important. For example, "Alex" has a hypersensitivity to auditory input. He was so distracted by the sound of a bumblebee buzzing around a bush 30 feet from the house that he couldn't stay on task to complete his chores. He repeatedly put his hands over his ears, trying to muffle the sound of the bumblebee.

With fixated attention the AS child becomes intensely preoccupied and selectively focused on an object or activity. Because of this fixated attention, they fail to attend to other stimuli (verbal information or interactions) in their environment. For example, Alex's teacher was reviewing plans for a class trip the next day. Alex's attention was so focused on the ducks printed on his teacher's tie that he failed to "hear" what his teacher was saying, and did not respond to the teacher's questions.

Anxiety Disorders and Depression

Anxiety and depression are more common among older AS children and adults (Klin, Volkmar, & Sparrow, 2000). As AS children mature, they become increasingly aware of how they differ from their peers, and the difficulty they have in social relationships. They are aware of "standards" of behavior and achievement which are difficult for them to attain. Frequently, as a result of these differences, the AS child becomes the victim of peer teasing or ostracizing. In response to these very real differences, taunting, and social consequences, the AS child may become depressed. Adolescent depression tends to manifest differently than in adults. Instead of expressed sadness or withdrawn behaviors, it is manifested through acting-out or an irritable demeanor.

If the AS child responds with anxious behaviors, it could manifest as nail-biting, tugging at clothing, hair pulling, avoidance of school or other social situations, etc. In some cases, the anxious behaviors may meet the criteria of an anxiety disorder such as social anxiety, or school phobia. Similarly, if the depression becomes chronic and significantly interferes with daily life, it may meet the criteria for a mood disorder. In a study by Klin et al. 2000, 15 percent of AS children had a co-existing mood disorder.

Distinguishing between anxious and depressed behaviors, which meet the criteria for a disorder is not easy and professional consultation is recommended. Generally, if the anxious or depressed behaviors are short-lasting, or are a normal response to an event, then the anxious or depressed behaviors should remit. If they are chronic, and significantly interfere with daily life, professional treatment may be needed.

Obsessive-Compulsive Disorder

Although OCD does occur in some individuals with AS (19 percent according to Klin et al. 2000), some features of AS can be mistaken for obsessive compulsive disorder: cognitive rigidity, rigid adherence to routines and schedules, and a restricted range of interests. For example, it is common for AS children and adults to have a consuming interest in a specific limited topic, e.g., trains, elevators, dinosaurs, and presidents of the United States. They typically develop extensive knowledge about their specific area of interest. What distinguishes behaviors associated with these interests from OCD is that the AS individual does not feel compelled to read about "trains" or "ride a train" as a means of reducing feelings of anxiety; they simply find pleasure in pursuing their area of interest. For example, Alex has a consuming interest in trains. He collects books, magazines, catalogues and videos about trains, train schedules, and model trains, and he knows the history of trains, how they are built, and frequently rides trains. However, he is able to go through the day without train-related activities interfering with his daily routines. Given the opportunity, however, to read a book, or talk about something he likes, he will inevitably discuss/read about trains.

Another feature of the AS child's restricted range of interests is that they are ego-syntonic, i.e., the AS youngster does not see anything wrong with engaging in the absorbing interest. An OCD youngster is generally bothered by the obsessive thoughts and compulsive behaviors and experiences them as intrusive and disruptive to his or her life, and is a source of anxiety.

Oppositional-Defiant Disorder

AS children can be difficult to manage, and exhibit noncompliant behaviors. However, the reasons for the apparent noncompliance are different. An important difference between an AS child and an oppositional-defiant child is volition. While the oppositional-defiant child will planfully disobey the "rules," the AS child will generally make an effort to follow the rules as he or she understands them. However, his or her understanding of the rule may be impaired either because of a miscommunication (comprehension or language pragmatics), sensory overload, misreading of contextual (nonverbal) cues, inattention, or because he or she acted impulsively. Additionally, when an AS child learns a rule in one environment, the behavior will not generalize to a new setting. In the new setting the contextual cues are different, and the AS child will perceive the similar setting/situation as entirely different.

Schizophrenia

Many aspects of AS can be confused with psychotic behavior. An untreated AS child can present as a solitary individual, uninterested in social interaction and intensely preoccupied with internal thoughts. Poor language pragmatic skills can contribute to a child verbalizing tangential thoughts that are loosely related to ongoing discussions. For example, when Alex was first enrolled in a therapeutic school, he had a history of many years of engaging in solitary activities. His parents reported that his behavior had become increasing unmanageable, and it became easier to allow him to entertain himself with his solitary activities, rather than endure his acting out behaviors when they tried to force him to interact with other family members. He spent many hours each day watching television, playing computer games, or using other electronic game equipment. When first confronted with new routines and adult interactions from which he could not escape, Alex retreated into his private mental world of television and computer game characters. He expressed fear of one of these characters, and often imagined "seeing" the character in his room at night. He was provisionally diagnosed with a psychotic disorder. But as "Alex" adapted to his new environment and routines, learned age-appropriate social skills, and improved his pragmatic language skills, he became more interactive with others, and there were no more occurrences of his "psychotic" behaviors.

Diagnostic Assessment

Developmental History and AS Screening Test

If a diagnosis of Asperger Syndrome has not yet been established, then assessment should begin with a developmental history and a screening test such as the Asperger Syndrome Diagnostic Scale (Myles, Bock, & Simpson, 2001), the Gilliam Autism Rating Scale (Gilliam, 1995), or the Childhood Autism Rating Scale (Schopler, Reichler, & Renner, 1988). A developmental history provides information about language, motor, and social milestones. Were these milestones met, or delayed, and, if delayed, how long? This information can be obtained through a structured parent interview such as the Autism Diagnostic Interview – Revised (Lord, Rutter, & Le Couteur, 1994). Also, questions contained in the Gilliam Autism Rating Scale elicit information about early childhood development, and can be used to develop further questions about the child's history.

Language Pragmatics

Although not yet listed as a diagnostic criterion in the DSM-IV, it is generally accepted that AS children have deficits in language pragmatics. Therefore, an assessment of pragmatic language skills would help to identify strengths and weakness in the practical use of language skills. The Pragmatic Language Survey (DuCharme, 1992) provides a thorough assessment of these skills. The Pragmatic Skills Survey assesses four categories of communication: topic, purpose, abstraction, and visual/gestural cues. The survey results provide a functional description of the student' s communication skills with adults, with peers, and in various settings.

Neuropsychological Testing

A diagnostic protocol for an AS child should also include a complete neuropsychological battery of tests to assess functioning in multiple areas:

attention, mental control, intellectual functioning, sensory perception and motor skills, auditory perception and memory, and visual perception and memory.

Attention and Mental Control

The focus of these tasks is to assess brief passive attention, short-term concentration skills, inhibition of routinized information, the ability to visualize and manipulate information in working memory, and the ability to shift cognition and behavior as task demands change. These tasks include reciting the alphabet, days of the week (forward and backward), and months of the year (forward and backward) (Bender, 1979), Serial Threes (counting forward (from 1) and backward (from 100) by threes, and spelling selected words forward and backward, Visual Continuous Performance task (Mesulam, 1985), Trail Making Test (Reitan, 1958), Verbal Fluency (FAS), and Wisconsin Card Sorting Test (Grant & Berg, 1948).

Intellectual Functioning

IQ assessment not only provides an overall assessment of intellectual skills but also differential assessment of verbal versus performance skills, processing speed, working memory. The Wechsler Intelligence Scale for Children, IV (Wechsler, 2003), or the Wechsler Adult Intelligence Scale, III (Wechsler, 1997a), provides a comprehensive assessment of intellectual functioning. Analysis of the subtests provides information about other areas that are relevant to a diagnosis of AS: knowledge of conventional social customs and social judgment, visual-motor skills, versus visual problem-solving without a motor component, executive functions (e.g., organizing, planning, sequencing, attention), and visual and auditory memory.

Visual-Spatial and Motor Skills

These tests assess the brain's ability to process and integrate visual and motor information (e.g., eye-hand coordination), visual reasoning without a motor component, the ability to organize and execute a drawing strategy, and spatial organization. These tests include IQ subtests (Block Design, Object Assembly, and Matrix Reasoning), Beery-Buktenica Developmental Test of Visual Motor Integration (Beery, 1989), Rey Osterrieth Complex Figure (Rey, 1941; Osterrieth, 1944; Meyers & Meyers, 1955), Benton Judgment of Line Orientation (Benton, Hannay, & Varnay, 1975), Rey Tangled Lines (Rey, 1964; Senior, Kelly & Salzman, 1999), Hooper Visual Organization Test (Hooper, 1958), and Draw a Clock (Goodglass & Kaplan, 1972).

Auditory and Visual Perception and Memory

These tests assess the brain's ability to process auditory information (language and non-language domains such as music) and visual information (written versus pictorial/abstract), and the ability to encode and recall it. The Wechsler Memory Scale, Third Edition (Wechsler, 1997b) includes multiple subtests which provide a comprehensive assessment of auditory perception and memory, as well as visual perception and memory. The ability to "hear" the prosodic quality of language is impaired in AS individuals. The Seashore Rhythms Test (Halstead, 1947) assesses non-language auditory perception skills. In this test the individual must discriminate between pairs of musical beats, some of which are the same and others, which are different.

Social Skill Assessment

Deficits in social skills are one of the salient characteristics of AS individuals. The Social Skills Rating Scale (Gresham & Elliott, 1990) has three forms (self, parent, and teacher) and assesses social skills in a variety of categories: cooperation, assertion, empathy, self-control, externalizing and internalizing behaviors, and academic competence. A comparison of the responses from student, parent, and teacher provides an overview of the student's self-assessment skills.

The diagnostic clarity of the criteria used for Asperger Syndrome needs to be improved. We have a working knowledge for a basis for improvement. Level of language skill and prosody, social adaptability, social pragmatic language, cognition, sensory motor integration, and maladaptive behavior are categorical aspects of Asperger Syndrome. These categories of behavior are most often referred to as component characteristics of a complete picture of the functioning of a person with an AS diagnosis.

The limitations of the diagnostic systems in current use complicate the process used to identify those in need of specialized services. It remains important to address the symptoms currently presented by individuals in need of services. And hopefully the revision of the DSM-IV in 2010 will result in an improved system for the depiction of a person with Asperger Syndrome.

References

Aman, C.J., Roberts, Jr., R.J., Pennington, B.F. (1998). A Neuropsychological Examination of the Underlying Deficit in Attention Deficit Hyperactivity Disorder: Frontal Lobe Versus Right Parietal Lobe Theories. *Developmental Psychology, 34*,5, 956–969.

American Psychiatric Association (1994). Diagnostic and statistical manual of mental disorders (4th ed.), Washington, DC: Author.

Asperger, H. (1944). Die 'autistischen Psychopathen' im Kindesalter, *Archiv fur Psychiatric und Nervenkrankheiten*, 117, 76–136. Translated by U. Frith (Ed.), *Autism and Asperger syndrome* (1991, pp. 37–92). Cambridge: Cambridge University Press.

Barnhill, G.P., Myles, B.S. (2001). Attributional style and depression in adolescents with Asperger syndrome. *Journal of Positive Behavior Interventions*, Sum 3(3), 175–182.

Barnhill, E. (2000). *Attributional style and depression in adolescents with Asperger Syndrome.* Unpublished doctoral dissertation, University of Kansas.

Barnhill, G.P. (2001). What's New in AS Research: A Synthesis of Research Conducted by the Apserger Syndrome Project. *Intervention in School and Clinic*, 36(5), 300–305.

Baron-Cohen, S., O'Riordan, M., Stone, V., Jones, R., Plaisted, K. (1999). Recognition of Faux Pas by Normally Developing Children and Children with Asperger Syndrome or High-Functioning Autism. *Journal of Autism and Developmental Disorders*, 29, 5.

Bender, M.B. (1979). Defects in reversal of serial order of symbols. *Neuropsychologia*, 17, 125–138.

Beery, K.E. (1989). *Revised administration, scoring, and teaching manual for the Developmenal Test of Visual-Motor Integration.* Cleveland, OH: Modern Curriculum Press.

Benton, A.L., & Hamsher, K. de S. (1976). *Multilngual Aphasia Examination.* Iowa City: University of Iowa.

Casanova, M.F., Buzhoeveden, D.P., Switala, A.E., & Roy, E. (2002). Asperger's syndrome and cortical neuropathology. *Journal of Child Neurology*, 17(2), 142–145.

Channon, S., Charman, T., Heap, J., Crawford, C., Rios, P. (2001). Real-life-type problem-solving in Asperger's syndrome. *Journal of Autism & Developmental Disorders*, 3(5), 461–469.

Courchesne, E., Townsend, J., Akshoomoff, N. A., Saitoh, O., Yeung Courchesne, R., Lincoln, A., Hector, E.J., Haas, R.H., Schreibman, L., Lau, L. (1994). Impairment in shifting attention in autistic and cerebellar patients. *Behavioral Neuroscience*, 108, 5, 848–865.

Craig, J., Baron-Cohen, S. (1999). Creativity and imagination in autism and Asperger syndrome. *Journal of Autism & Developmental Disorders*, Aug 29, 4, 314–326.

de Leon, M.J., Munoz, R.J., Pieo, S.E. (1986). Is there a right-hemisphere dysfunction in Asperger's syndrome? *British Journal of Psychiatry*, Jun 148, 745–756.

Dewey, M. (1991). Living with Asperger's syndrome. In Frith, Uta (Ed). *Autism and Asperger syndrome*, (pp. 184–206). New York, NY, US: Cambridge University Press.

Dyer, K., Kneringer, M.J., Luce, S.C. (1996). An efficient method of ensuring program quality for adults with developmental disabilities in community- based apartments. *Consulting Psychology Journal: Practice & Research*, Sum 48(3), 171.

DuCharme, R.W. (1992). *The Learning Clinic Pragmatic Language Survey.* Brooklyn, CT: The Learning Clinic.

DuCharme, R.W., McGrady, K. (2003). *Promoting the Healthy Development of Children with Asperger Syndrome: Education & Life Skills Issues.* Connecticut College, New London, CT.

Dunn, W., Myles, B.S., & Orr, S. (2002). Sensory processing issues associated with Asperger Syndrome: A preliminary investigation. *The American Journal of Occupational Therapy*, 56(1), 97–102.

Ehlers, S., Gillberg, C. (1993). The epidemiology of Asperger syndrome: A total population study. *Journal of Child Psychology & Psychiatry & Allied Disciplines*, Nov 34(8), 1327–1350.

Ehlers, S., Nyden, A., Gillberg, C., Dahlgren, S., Annika, et al. (1997). Asperger syndrome, autism and attention disorders: A comparative study of the cognitive profiles of 120 children. *Journal of Child Psychology & Psychiatry & Allied Disciplines*, Feb 38(2), 207–217.

Ehlers, S., Gillberg, C., Wing, L. (1999). Autistic Spectrum Screening Questionnaire (ASSQ). *Journal of Autism & Developmental Disorders.*

Eisenmajer, R., Prior, M., Leekham, S., Wing, L., et al. (1996). Comparison of clinical symptoms in autism and Asperger's disorder. *Journal of the Academy of Child & Adolescent Psychiatry,* Nov 35(11), 1523–1531.

Frith, U. (1991). *Autism and Asperger syndrome.* New York: Cambridge University Press.

Frith, U., Happe, F. (1994). Autism: Beyond "theory of mind." *Cognition, 50,* 115–132.

Ghaziuddin, M., Butler, E., Tsai, L., Ghaziuddin, N. (1994). Is clumsiness a marker for Asperger syndrome? *Journal of Intellectual Disability Research,* Oct, 38(5), 519–527.

Ghaziuddin, M., Butler, E. (1998). Clumsiness in autism and Asperger syndrome: A further report. *Journal of Intellectual Disability Research,* Feb 42(1), 43–48.

Gilchrist, A., Green, J., Cox, A., Burton, D., Rutter, M., Le Couteur, A. (2001). Development and current functioning in adolescents with Asperger syndrome: A comparative study. *Journal of Child Psychology & Pscyhiatry & Allied Disciplines.*

Gillberg, C. (1993). Asperger syndrome and clumsiness. *Journal of Autism & Develomental Disorders,* Dec 23(4), 686–687.

Gillberg, C. (1995). *Clinical Child Neuropsychiatry.* Cambridge and New York: Cambridge University Press.

Gilliam, J.E. (1995). *Gilliam Autism Rating Scale.* Austen, TX: Pro-Ed, Inc.

Goodglass, H., & Kaplan, E. (1972). *The Assessment of Aphasia and Related Disorders.* Philadelphia: Lea & Fibiger.

Grant, D.A., & Berg, E.A. (1948). A behavioral analysis of degree of reinforcement and ease of shifting to new responses in a Weigle-type card sorting problem. *Journal of Experimental Psychology, 32,* 404–411.

Green, D., Baird, G., Barnett, A.L., Henderson, L., Huber, J., Henderson, S.E. (2002). The severity and nature of motor impairment in Asperger's syndrome: A comparison with Specific Developmental Disorders of Motor Function. *Journal of Child Psychology & Psychiatry & Allied Disciplines,* Jun 43(5), 655–668.

Gresham, F.M. & Elliott, S.N. (1990). *Social Skills Rating System.* Circle Pines, MN: American Guidance Service.

Grossman, J.B., Klin, A., Carter, A.S., Volkmar, F.R. (2000). Verbal bias in recognition of facial emotions in children with Asperger Syndrome. *Journal of Child Psychology & Psychiatry & Applied Disciplines.*

Halstead, W.C. (1947). *Brain and Intelligence.* Chicago: University of Chicago Press.

Happe, F.G.E. (1995). The role of age and verbal ability in the theory of mind task performance of subjects with autism. *Child Development, 66,* 843–855.

Hooper, H.E. (1958). *The Hooper Visual Organization Test.* Manual. Beverly Hills, CA: Western Psychological Services.

Jolliffe, T., Baron-Cohen, S. (2000). Linguistic processing in high-functioning adults with autism or Asperger's syndrome. Is global coherence impaired? *Psychological Medicine, 30,* 1169–1187.

Kanner, L. (1943). Autistic disturbance of affective contact. *Nervous Child, 2,* 217–250.

Klin, A., Volkmar, F., & Sparrow, S. (2000). *Asperger Syndrome.* New York, NY: The Guilford Press.

Klin, A., Volkmar, F.R. (1997). Asperger's syndrome. In D.J. Cohen & F.R. Volkmar (Eds), *Handbook of autism and pervasive developmental disorders* (2nd ed., pp 94–112). New York: Wiley.

Klin, A., Volkmar, F.R., Sparrow, S.S., Cicchetti, D.V. (1995). Validity and neuropsychological characterization of Asperger Syndrome: Convergence with Nonverbal Learning Disabilities syndrome. *Journal of Child Psychology & Psychiatry & Applied Disciplines,* 1127–1140.

Leekham, S., Libby, S., Wing, L., Gould, J., Gillberg, C. (2000). Comparison of ICD-10 and Gillberg's Criteria for Asperger Syndrome. *Autism: The International Journal of Research and Practice*, *4*, 85–100. This was in the abstract: "ICD-10 & Diagnostic Interview for Social & Communication Disorders". (DISCO)

Lord, C., Rutter, M. & Le Couteur, A. (1994). Autism Diagnostic Interview Revised: A revised version of a diagnostic interview for caregivers of individuals with possible pervasive developmental disorders. *Journal of Autism and Developmental Disorders, 24*(5), 659–685.

Manjiviona, J., Prior, M. (1999). Neuropsychological profiles of children with Asperger syndrome and autism. *Autism*. Dec, *3*, 4, 327–356.

Matthews, A. (1996). Employment training and the development of a support model within employment for adults who experience Asperger syndrome and autism: The Gloucestershire Group Homes Model. *In Morgan, H. Adults with autism: A guide to theory and practice.* 163–184. New York, NY, US: Cambridge University Press.

Mawhood, L., Howlin, P. (1999). The outcome of a supported employment scheme for high-functioning adults with autism or Asperger syndrome. *Autism*, Sep 3(3), 229–254.

Mesibov, G.B., Shea, V., & Adams, L.W. (2001). *Understanding Asperger Syndrome and High Functioning Autism.* New York: Kluwer Academic/Plenum Publishers.

Mesulam, M.-M. (1985). *Principles of Behavioral Neurology.* Philadelphia: F.A. Davis.

Meyers, J., & Meyers, K. (1955). *The Meyers Scoring System for the Rey Complex Figure and the Recognition Trial: Professional Manual.* Odessa, FL: Psychological Assessment Resources.

Minshew, N.J., Goldstein, G., Siegel, D.J. (1995). Speech and language in high-functioning autistic individuals. *Neuropsychology*, April 9(2) 255–261.

Miyahara, M., Tsujii, M., Hori, M., Nakanishi, K., Kageyama, H., Sugiyama, T. (1997). Motor incoordination in children with Asperger syndrome and learning disabilities. *Journal of Autism & Developmental Disorders*, Oct, *27*(5), 595–603.

Morris, R.G., Rowe, A., Fox, N., Feigenbaum, J.D., Miotto, E.C., Howlin, (1999). Spatial working memory in Aspeger's syndrome and in patients with focal frontal and temporal lobe lesions. *Brain & Cognition.*

Myles, B.S., Bock, S.J., & Simpson, R.L. (2001). *Asperger Syndrome Diagnostic Scale.* Austen, TX: Pro-Ed, Inc.

Nesbitt, S. (2000). Why and why not? Factors influencing employment for individuals with Asperger syndrome. *Austim*, Dec 4(4), 357–369.

Osterrieth, P.A. (1944). Le test de copie d'une figure complex: Contribution l'etude de la perception et de la memoire. *Archives de Psychologie, 30*, 286–356.

Ozonoff, S., South, M., & Miller, J. (2000). DSM-IV defined Asperger syndrome: cognitive, behavioral and early history differentiation from high-functioning autism. *Autism: The International Journal of Research and Practice, 4*, 29–46.

Perner, J., & Wimmer, H. (1985). "John thinks that Mary thinks that . . . " Attribution of second-order beliefs by 5–10 year old children. *Journal of Experimental Child Psychology, 39*, 437–471.

Raja, M., Azzoni, A. (2001). Asperger's disorder in the emergency psychiatric setting. *General Hospital Psychiatry, 23*, 285–293.

Reitan, R.M. (1958). Validity of the Trail Making Test as an indication of organic brain damage. *Perceptual and Motor Skills, 8*, 271.

Rey, A. (1941). L'examen psychologique dans les cas d'encephalopathie traumatique. *Archives de Pschologie, 28*, 286–340.

Rey, A. (1964). *L'examen clinique en psychologie.* Paris: Presses Universitaires de France.

Rourke, B.P., Fisk, J.L., & Strang, J.D. (1983). *Child neurophyschology: An introduction to theory, research, and clinical practice.* New York: Guilford Press.

Rourke, B.P. (1995). *Syndrome of Nonverbal Learning Disabilities.* New York: Guilford Press.

Schopler, E., Mesibov, G.B., & Kunce, L.J. (1998). *Asperger Syndrome or High-functioning Autism?* New York, NY: Plenum Press.

Schopler, E., Reichler, R.J., & Renner, B.R. (1988). *The Childhood Autism Rating Scale (CARS).* Los Angeles: Western Psychological Services.

Schultz, R.T., Romanski, L.M., Tsatsanis, K.D. (2000). Neurofunctional models of autistic disorder and Asperger syndrome: Clues from neuroimaging. *In Klin, Ami (Ed); Volkmar, Fred R. (Ed); et al. Asperger syndrome. (pp. 172–209).*

Scott, F.J., Baron-Cohen, S., Bolton, P., Brayne, C. (2002). *The CAST (Childhood Asperger Syndrome Test).* Sage Publications and The National Autistic Society, 6(1), 9–31.

Senior, G., Kelly, M., Salzman, L. (1999). *Clinical utility of the Rey Tangled Lines Test.* Poster session presented at the 19th Annual National Academy of Neuropsychology Conference, San Antonio, TX, November 10–13, 1999.

Shriberg, L.D., Paul, R., McSweeny, J.L., Klin, A., Cohen, D.J. (2001). Speech and prosody characteristics of adolescents and adults with high-functioning autism and Aspeger syndrome. *Journal of Speech, Language, & Hearing Research,* Oct 44(5), 1097–1115.

Shulman, C., Yirmiya, N., Greenbaum, C.W. (1995). From categorization to classification: A comparison among individuals with a retardation, and normal development. *Journal of Abnormal Psychology,* Nov 104(4), 601–609.

Szatmari, P., Bartolucci, G., Bremner, R. (1989). Asperger's syndrome and autism: Comparison of early history and outcome. *Developmental Medicine & Child Neurology,* Dec, 31, 6, 709–720.

Tantam, D. (1988). Asperger's syndrome: annotation. *Journal of Child Psychology and Psychiatry. 29,* 245–255.

Tantam, D. (2000). Adolescence and adulthood of Individuals with Asperger Syndrome. *Asperger Syndrome,* 367–399.

Tonge, B.J., Brereton, A.V., Gray, K.M., Einfeld, S.L. (1999). Behavioural and emotional disturbance in high-functioning autism and Asperger syndrome. *Autism,* Jun 3(2), 117–130.

Volkmar, F.R., Klin, A., Pauls, D. (1998). Nosological and Genetic Aspects of Asperger Syndrome. *Journal of Autism and Developmental Disorders,* 28(5), 457–463.

Wechsler, D. (1997a). *Manual for the Wechsler Adult Intelligence Scale, Third edition.* San Antonio, TX: Psychological Corporation.

Wechsler, D. (1997b). *Wechsler Memory Scale,* Third Edition. San Antonio, TX: The Psychological Corporation.

Wechsler, D. (2003). *Manual for the Wechsler Intelligence Scale for Children, Fourth edition.* San Antonio, TX: Psychological Corporation.

Weimer, A.K., Schatz, A.M., Lincoln, A., Ballantyne, A.O., Trauner, D.A. (2001). "Motor" impairment in Asperger Syndrome: Evidence for a deficit in proprioception. *Journal of Developmental & Behavioral Pediatrics,* Apr 22(2), 92–101. Wing, L. (1993). The definition and prevalence of autism: A review. *European Child and Adolescent Psychiatry, 2,* 61–74.

World Health Organization. (1992). *International Classification of diseases* (10th ed.). (ICD-10) Geneva, Switzerland: Author.

Chapter 2

Social Skills Instruction for Children with Asperger Syndrome

Brenda Smith Myles

Although relatively little research has been conducted on the nature of the social disability in Asperger Syndrome (AS) (Klin, Volkmar, & Sparrow, 2000; Myles & Simpson, 2002), researchers and practitioners generally agree that this area presents the greatest challenge throughout life (Barnhill, Hagiwara, Myles, Simpson, Brick, & Griswold, 2000; Church, Alisanski, & Amanullah, 2000; Myles & Adreon, 2001; Szatmari, 1991; Williams, 2001). The impact of social skills difficulties is pervasive across varying environments, even in structured settings designed to elicit prosocial behaviors. Social skills challenges range from not being able to develop and keep friendships to being ridiculed by peers to not being able to keep a job due to a lack of understanding of workplace culture and relationships among subordinates and supervisors (Baron-Cohen, O'Riordan, Stone, Jones, & Plaisted, 1999; MacLeod, 1999; Myles & Simpson, 2003).

Despite their importance, few studies have been published on interventions that can address the myriad of social issues affecting children and youth with AS. The studies that have been conducted have had varying success in helping children and youth with AS acquire social skills (Bledsoe, Myles, & Simpson, 2003; Barnhill, Cook, Tebbenkamp, & Myles, 2002; Howlin & Yates; 1999; Marriage, Gordon, & Brand, 1995; Rogers & Myles, 2001). Although each of these authors approached social skills in a different manner, they shared a recurring theme—emphasis was placed on supporting and developing skills rather than trying to eliminate inappropriate skills through behavior reduction procedures. In addition, all of the strategies are cognitively based. They focus on explaining to the individual when a specific strategy is needed, how it can be used and why it is needed. Cognitively based strategies appear effective in the social (Barnhill et al., 2002; Bledsoe et al., in press; Howlin & Yates, 1999; Marriage et al., 1995; Rogers & Myles, 2001), emotional (Hare, 1997) and academic realms (Ben-Arieh, Myles, & Carlson, in press).

Social Supports that Facilitate Social Success

The pervasiveness of social deficits in AS demands a complex approach to social skills support. A three-tier program of social development has been proposed as a means to address this area. Each of these components is intricately combined and all three are equally necessary. The first element in the program is instruction or directly teaching the child or youth with AS essential social skills. The second phase of social support is interpretation. Interpretation typically takes place after a specific social skill problem has occurred and includes strategies that aid the child in understanding that problem. The final element in social skills development is coaching—cueing the individual with AS to use the skills he has learned during instruction and interpretation (Myles & Adreon, 2001; Myles & Southwick, 1999). The purpose of this chapter is to describe each of these social support elements and overview specific strategies that can be used during each of the three phases.

Social Skills Instruction

Children and youth must be directly taught social skills they need to be successful. Targeting of social skills for instruction requires that an assessment of social skills be conducted. Observation of social skills use in natural environments as well as student, teacher, and parent completion of social skills scales and functional behaviors assessments can provide this information (Goldstein & McGinnis, 1997; Lewis, Scott, & Sugai, 1994). Instructional procedures include (a) direct instruction, (b) acting lessons, (c) the Power Card strategy, (c) social stories, and (d) conflict resolution.

DIRECT INSTRUCTION. The instructional sequence that facilitates learning of social skills includes: (a) rationale, (b) presentation, (c) modeling, (d) verification, (e) evaluation, and (f) generalization. In order for social skills instruction to be effective with children and youth with AS they need to understand the *rationale*—why concepts required for mastery are relevant and how they fit with the knowledge they already have. That is, the rationale for a social skill should include (a) why the information is useful, (b) how the individual can use the information, and (c) where it fits in with the knowledge he already possesses. The *presentation* should be active and multimodal encouraging children not only to listen and/or view content, but also to respond to questions, share observations, and provide and receive meaningful corrective feedback. Direct instruction does *not* mean presenting a worksheet and telling the child or youth to follow the directions. *Modeling* follows presentation. During *modeling* the child is shown what to do by the instructor. The model should be presented frequently, with the context for its use clearly spelled out. One common mistake must be avoided: We often tell children and youth with AS what *not* to do without providing the alternative—what they are supposed to do. Generally, it is preferable not to present negative modeling or showing the student how "not" to engage in the behavior appropriately because the student may focus on the misapplication of the behavior and attempt to use these negative skills. At the *verification* stage, the therapist closely monitors the child's understanding of what is being taught and his emotional state, providing opportunities for students to practice the skill in a controlled setting. Social skills acquisition requires *evaluation* from both the adult and the child with AS. A variety of methods should be employed to assess the child's understanding and use of the skill. For example, children with AS should self-evaluate their skill performance and set goals for generalization and skill maintenance. Finally, *generalization* programming should be a part of each lesson. Opportunities for the individual with AS to use newly acquired social skills in a variety of settings and structures (i.e., lunch, music, recess) must be provided. Assistance from parents is also invaluable to ensure generalization as they can set up and/or observe home- and community-based events in which the youth is expected to use the skill. Parents, depending on their time constraints, knowledge on how to observe and provide feedback, or level of social understanding may require different levels of support in helping their children with AS generalize social skills (Myles & Simpson, 2003).

ACTING LESSONS.   Many adults with AS recommend acting lessons to teach social skills. Acting lessons teach persons with AS how to express emotions that are context specific as well as how to interpret others' emotions, feelings, and voices. Acting lessons contain several direct instruction components (i.e., modeling, simulation and feedback). Perhaps the most important elements of this approach are (a) practice in a positive environment and (b) acknowledgement that everyone, not only individuals with AS, require some sort of social practice (Myles & Adreon, 2001; Myles & Southwick, 1999).

THE POWER CARD STRATEGY.   The Power Card is a visual aid that uses a child's special interest to help her understand social situations, routines, the meaning of language, and the hidden curriculum (Gagnon, 2001). This intervention contains two components: a script and the Power Card. A therapist, teacher or parent develops a brief script written at the child's comprehension level detailing the problem situation or target behavior that includes a description of the behavior and describes how the child's special interest has addressed that social challenge. This solution is then generalized back to the child. The Power Card, the size of a business card or trading card, contains a picture of the special interest and a summary of the solution that is portable to promote generalization. The Power Card can be carried or it can be velcroed inside a book, notebook, or locker. It may also be placed on the corner of a child's desk (Gagnon, 2001). This strategy has been empirically investigated with two children. In one case, the Power Card strategy resulted in marked behavior change and general-ization across settings; a second child experienced moderate success when the Power Card strategy was used (Myles, Keeling, & Van Horn, 2001). Figure 1 provides a sample script and Power Card used to help Jennifer, an eight-year old girl, to remember to wash her hands. Jennifer's special interest was Angelica from the *Rugrats*.

The Power Card strategy is not appropriate for every child or for every situation. Table 1 overviews situations and behaviors for which the strategy may or may not be appropriate.

SOCIAL STORIES.   According to Gray (1995), a social story is designed to assist individuals in understanding and appropriately following social protocol. Guidelines for writing social stories address salient elements of a given social situation, including who, what, when, where, and why (Gray, 2000; Gray & Garand, 1993). Within this prescriptive framework, social stories are individualized to specific situations, and to individuals of vary-ing abilities and lifestyles. Social stories may exclusively be written docu-ments or paired with pictures, audio-tapes, or video-tapes (Swaggart et al., 1995). They may be created by educators, mental health professionals, and parents, often with student input. The basic social story formula generally consists of four types of sentences: (a) descriptive, (b) directive, (c) perspec-tive, and (d) affirmative (Gray, 2000). *Descriptive sentences* define a social setting and what people typically do in a particular situation. *Directive sen-tences* guide an individual to engage in an appropriate response in a defined situation and often begin with *I will work on, I will try,* or *I have a choice, I may. Perspective sentences* refer to the internal status of the person for whom the social story is written. Finally, *affirmative sentences* express a shared

Angelica Says, "Wash Those Hands"

by Rachele M. Hill

Angelica knows how important it is to keep hands clean. She does not want to catch any yucky germs from "those babies!" Germs can cause coughing, sneezing, and runny noses. Angelica definitely does not want to catch a cold! She washes her hands often and always after using the bathroom. She knows that washing her hands helps her from catching a cold.

Angelica wants you to have clean hands, too. She wants you to remember to wash your hands often and every time after you go to the bathroom.

Angelica wants you to remember these three things:

- Wash your hands after you go to the bathroom.
- Always use soap.
- Dry your hands completely.

Angelica can be very bossy, but she does have manners when it comes to having clean hands. Angelica says, "Please wash your hands!"

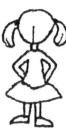

- Wash your hands after go to the bathroom.
- Always use soap.
- Dry your hands comple

Figure 1. Sample script and Power Card. (*Source*: E. Gagnon, (2001). *The Power Card strategy: Using special interests to motivate children and youth with Asperger Syndrome and autism.* Shawnee Mission, KS: Autism Asperger Publishing Company)

opinion or value. Although social stories have gained widespread recognition and popularity (Myles & Simpson, 2001), only two studies have been designed to measure the efficacy of using this strategy with individuals with AS (Rogers & Myles, 2001; Bledsoe et al., in press). Both investigations, however, resulted in behavior change. Figure 2 contains a social story that was successfully used to modify the etiquette of an adolescent with AS (Bledsoe et al., 2003).

**Table 1. Situations and Behaviors for Which the Power Card Strategy
May or May Not Be Appropriate**

The Power Card Strategy is appropriate for behaviors or situations in which:

- The student lacks understanding of what she is to do, such as hidden curriculum items, routines, or language use that the student has not been taught.
- The student does not understand that he has choices.
- The student has difficulty understanding that there is a cause-and-effect relationship between a specific behavior and its consequence.
- The student has difficulty remembering what to do without a prompt.
- The student does not understand the perspective of others.
- The student knows what to do when calm but cannot follow a given routine under stress.
- The student needs a visual reminder to recall the behavioral expectation for a situation.
- The student has difficulty generalizing.
- The student is difficult to motivate and may be motivated *only* by the special interest.
- The student has difficulty accepting direction from an adult.

The Power Card Strategy is usually *not* appropriate when:

- The student has sensory needs such as difficulty tolerating certain noises, smells or tastes. Although the strategy can help students realize that they may be experiencing a need for sensory input, it alone will not satisfy that need. The strategy may serve as a slight delay, however, by reminding the child what she needs to do to get her needs met.
- The child is extremely challenged cognitively and appears not to understand spoken language at the sentence or paragraph level. To use the Power Card Strategy, the child does not *have* to be a reader if pictures or graphics are used to explain the problem situation or behavior and the teacher serves as the reader.
- The student engages in the problem behavior only once. It is difficult to determine a cause or motivation for behavior unless it occurs somewhat frequently.
- The teacher or other adults do not have a positive relationship with the child. Remember, the Power Card Strategy is not a punishment. It should not be perceived as negative in any way. It is fulfilling a need for the child while capitalizing on his special interest.
- The child is in crisis. When the child is in the rage stage (Myles & Southwick, 1999), this technique will not work. Since the child is not functioning at his optimal level, he cannot make rationale decisions. Worse, yet, using the Power Card Strategy at the rage stage will make this technique less effective at times when it is otherwise appropriate.
- The child does not have a well-developed area of interest. In order to buy into the strategy, the child needs to want to follow the hero's directions.

Source: E. Gagnon (2001). *The Power Card strategy: Using special interests to motivate children and youth with Asperger Syndrome and autism.* Shawnee Mission, KS: Autism Asperger Publishing Company.

Cover page text:
Table Manners

Page 1 text:

Sometimes I like to sit with my friends and eat lunch.
We talk about lots of things like movies, music and video games.

Page 2 text:

I have noticed that my friends eat slowly and carefully to get their food and drink into their mouth.
They often wipe their mouth with a napkin while eating.
This keeps their clothes and table area neat and their mouth stays clean while they are eating.

Page 3 text:

I will try to eat slowly and carefully to get my food and drink into my mouth.
I can use a napkin to wipe off my mouth often while I eat.
If I do this, my friends will want to sit and talk to me at lunch.

Figure 2. Sample social story. (*Source*: R., Bledsoe, B. S., Myles, & R. L. Simpson, (2003). Use of a social story intervention to improve mealtime skills of an adolescent with Asperger Syndrome. *Autism, 7*, 289–295)

CONFLICT RESOLUTION.   As discussed throughout this book, children and youth with AS, encounter difficulties when faced with a problem or novel situation that does not readily present with a solution. Their primary response is often a meltdown, tantrum, refusal, or withdrawal. A understanding of and strategies for carrying out conflict resolution skills as presented in *Asperger Syndrome and Getting Along: A Conflict Resolution Program* (Keys, Trautman, & Mehaffey, in press) helps individuals with AS successfully master their environment without behavioral strife. Keys et al. curricula provides hands-on activities in the following areas: (a) understanding communication basics, (b) stress and what to do about it, (c) cooperating with others, (d) thinking differently about the same thing, (e) getting and receiving help, and (f) solving problems. The philosophy behind this curriculum is that self-understanding and personal problem solving precede empowering self to act on the outside environment.

Interpretation

No matter how much social skills instruction is provided to individuals with AS, some situations will occur that he does not understand. In these cases, the child or adolescent with AS requires a social interpreter—someone who can turn a confusing event into a meaningful interaction through explanation and clarification. Although criteria for social interpreters has not been empirically validated, it is generally accepted that these individuals (a) should have an understanding of AS and the child, in particular; (b) have an established rapport with the individual as well as an appreciation for the child's way of viewing the world; (c) enjoy working with the individual and voice that enjoyment; (d) indicate that learning is mutual; (e) work as an unobtrusive facilitator rather than as a dictator; (f) provide nonthreatening feedback; and (g) do not lecture, but provides general direction as needed (Myles & Adrcon, 2001; Myles & Simpson, 2003). Six strategies can be effective in interpreting social situations: (a) cartooning; (b) social autopsies; (c) the Situation, Options, Consequences, Choices, Strategies, Simulation (SOCCSS) strategy; (d) Stop, Observe, Deliberate, and Act (SODA), and (e) sensory awareness.

CARTOONING.   Visual symbols such as those found in cartoons may enhance social understanding by turning abstract and elusive events into something tangible and static that can be reflected upon (Hagiwara & Myles, 1999; Kuttler, Myles, & Carlson, 1998). Used as a generic term, cartooning has been implemented by speech/language pathologists for many years to enhance understanding in their clients. Several interventions use cartoon figures as an instructional medium: comic strip conversations (Gray, 2000), mind-reading (Howlin, Baron-Cohen, & Hadwin, 1999), and pragmaticism (Arwood & Brown, 1999). Two studies have been conducted on cartooning, both approaching the subject in different ways with positive finds. Parsons and Mitchell (1999) conducted a study that found that children with autism spectrum disorders could understand the role of thought bubbles in cartoons. A second study revealed that comic strip conversations were effective with an adolescent with AS (Rogers & Myles, 2001). The cartoon from this study appears in Figure 3.

SOCIAL AUTOPSIES.   Lavoie (cited in Bieber, 1994) developed social autopsies as a supportive and positive intervention to help children and youth understand social errors. A social autopsy occurs when an adult and child with AS analyze a specific social situation by identifying the social error, determining who may have been harmed by the error, deciding how to amend the situation, and creating a plan to prevent its reoccurrence. Lavoie recommends that every adult with whom the person with AS has regular contact, such as parents, teachers, and therapists, know how to do a social autopsy. Originally designed by LaVoie (cited in Bieber, 1994) to be a verbal strategy, the technique has been modified to include a worksheet to enhance child learning (see Figure 4).

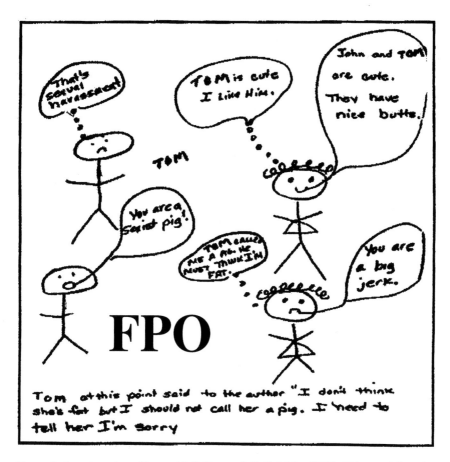

Figure 3. Sample cartoon.(*Source*: M. F. Rogers & B. S. Myles (2001). Using social stories and comic strip conversations to interpret social situations for an adolescent with Asperger Syndrome. *Intervention in School and Clinic, 36*, 310–313)

SITUATION, OPTIONS, CONSEQUENCES, CHOICES, STRATEGIES, SIMULATION **(SOCCSS).** SOCCSS provides an extensive analysis of social interactions by helping individuals with AS learn choice making, cause effect relationship, and problem-solving (Roosa, 1995). This adult-directed strategy helps children and youth with AS logically work through the situations by defining (a) the problem situation, (b) options the child may have in how to respond to that situation, and (c) consequences that would logically follow each options. The youth is then supported in making a choice among the options that were generated and developing a strategy to implement that choice. Finally, the child practices or simulates the strategy to ensure that

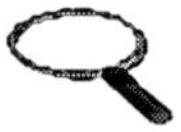

What happened? _____

_____

_____

_____

What was the social error?	Who was hurt by the social error?

What should be done to correct the error? _____

_____

_____

What could be done next time? _____

_____

_____

_____

_____

_____

_____

Figure 4. Social autopsies worksheet. (*Source*: B. S. Myles, & D. Adreon (2001). *Asperger Syndrome and adolescence: Practical solutions for school success*. Shawnee Mission, KS: Autism Asperger Publishing Company)

Table 2. SOCCSS Strategy Steps

- *Situation*: After a social problem occurs, the adult helps the child to define the situation. At first the adult will assume an active role in prompting and identifying, when necessary, answers to these questions. The goal, however, is for individual independence.
- *Options*: The adult and child brainstorm several options she might have chosen in the situation. All responses are accepted without evaluation. Initially, the adult may have to encourage the youth with AS to identify more than one option.
- *Consequences*: For each option generated, a consequence is listed. The adult prompts the child to respond to the question, "So what would happen if you... (*name the option*)?" Some options may have more than one consequence. Because it may be difficult for individuals with AS to understand cause and effect, role-play at this stage can serve as a prompt in identifying consequences.
- *Choices*: Options and consequences are prioritized. Following prioritization, the child is prompted to select the option that (a) appears doable and (b) will most likely help the child obtain personal wants or needs.
- *Strategies*: A plan is developed to carry out the *option* if the *situation* occurs. Although the adult and child may collaborate developing the strategy, the child should ultimately generate the plan to ensure a feeling of ownership and commitment to use the strategy.
- *Simulation*: The adult and child simulate the strategy: (a) using imagery, (b) talking with another about the plan, (c) writing down the plan, or (d) role-playing. Simulation should provide the individual with AS with the skills and confidence to carry out the plan.

Source: B. S. Myles & D. Adreon (2001). *Asperger Syndrome and adolescence: Practical solutions for school success*. Shawnee Mission, KS: Autism Asperger Publishing Company.

he could actually carry out his choice in a social setting. Table 2 provides further details on the steps of the SOCCSS strategy. Although designed as interpretive, this strategy can also be used as an instructional strategy. For example, therapists or teachers can identify problems that children with AS are likely to encounter and address them using SOCCSS so that the individuals with AS have a plan prior to a situation occurring (Myles & Simpson, 2001).

STOP, OBSERVE, DELIBERATE, AND ACT (SODA).   Similar to the SOCCSS strategy (Roosa, 1995), SODA is a visual, problem solving rubric that children and youth with AS can use to navigate unfamiliar social situations (Bock, 2001). It was designed as a multipurpose strategy that individuals with AS could use in almost any social gathering. (See Table 3.) SODA attempts to develop a schema for the child to understand novel environments and be an active decision-maker in determining how she will fit in. Bock has created the following series of questions about salient environmental factors that individuals with AS should ask themselves at each stage of SODA.

Stop: What is the room arrangement?, What is the activity or routine?, Where should I go to observe?

Table 3. SODA Strategy Steps

- *Stop*: During this step, the child with AS attempts to define the activities and their order as well as to identify a location near the activities from which he can observe the scene. The selected location should be one in which the child or youth can observe and learn information that will help him participate in the activity successfully.
- *Observe*: The observation period includes many facets that help the individual with AS create a schema: length of conversations, number of individuals involved in conversations, tone of conversations (i.e., formal, casual), strategies used to begin and end conversations, nonverbal language, and any routines that may be in place.
- *Deliberate*: Deliberation helps the child or youth develop an action plan. Depending on the situation, he may decide on a topic of conversation, quickly review social skills etiquette that would help him be successful (i.e., nonverbal cues, posture, social distance). Also included in this step is thoughtful deliberation on what others will think of him if he does or does not follow the social protocol he has observed.
- *Act*: The final stage of SODA includes participation in the social event using the strategies he identified during the deliberation stage. The *Act* stage also allows the individual to generalize skills that he may have learned in another setting.

Source: B. S. Myles & D. Adreon (2001). *Asperger Syndrome and adolescence: Practical solutions for school success.* Shawnee Mission, KS: Autism Asperger Publishing Company.

> *Observe:* What are the people doing?, What are the people saying?, What is the length of a typical conversation, What do the people do after they've visited?
>
> *Deliberate:* What would I like to do?, What would I like to say?, How will I know when others would like to visit longer **or** would like to end this conversation?
>
> *Act:* Approach person(s) with whom I'd like to visit., Say, "Hello, how are you?", Listen to person(s) **and** ask related questions., Look for cues that this person would like to visit longer **or** would like to end this conversation., End the conversation and walk away (see Table 3 for an elaboration on these steps).

SODA has been used successfully with eight students with AS (Bock, 2002). This strategy can be successful, but relies heavily on good social skills instruction. That is, the students using SODA should have the social skills required to execute each of the stages of the strategy.

SENSORY AWARENESS.   All the information we receive from the environment comes through our sensory systems. These seven systems serve as interpreters of incoming stimuli and are instrumental in how we act in our many environments. Thus, our visual, auditory, proprioceptive, vestibular, olfactory, and gustatory systems impact learning (Ayres, 1979; Dunn, 1999). Research has shown that the majority of individuals with AS have sensory integration problems (Dunn, Myles, & Orr, 2002; Myles, Cook, Miller, Rinner, & Robbins, 2000) that require direct assistance. This research has shown that each of the sensory systems is impaired in children and youth with AS and often the degree of impairment is similar to individuals with autism who have IQs in the cognitively challenged range. Several programs appear effective in meeting the sensory needs of children and youth with AS. Among them are (a) *Asperger Syndrome and Sensory Issues: Practical Solutions for Making Sense of the World* (Myles et al., 2000); (b) *Building Bridges Through Sensory Integration* (Yack, Sutton, & Aquilla, 1998); and (c) *The Tool Chest for Teachers, Parents, and Students* (Henry Occupational Therapy Services, Inc., 1998).

SELF-AWARENESS.   Self-awareness often begins with self-understanding. The book *What Is Asperger Syndrome, and How Will It Affect Me? A Guide for Young People* (Ives, 2001) helps young people to understand their AS. It acknowledges that it is often difficult to explain AS to others and that people will generally not be able to tell if he has AS just by looking at him. The book sends a positive yet realistic message to children and youth. Ives (2001) concludes the book with these statements to young people with AS:

> It is important to remember that you are not alone. There are many people with Asperger syndrome. People with Asperger syndrome can go on to achieve a lot of things, including going to a university, getting a good job, living in their own house. You will always have Asperger syndrome although, as time goes on, you may get better at things you used to find really hard. . . . Most importantly, remember that you are exactly the same person you always were, before you ever heard the words Asperger syndrome. Only now you have a way of understanding why you find some things tricky, and also can find ways of making life easier for yourself (p. 20).

Self-understanding also includes the ability to read and self-monitor positive and negative reactions. Children and youth with AS, however, often have difficulty with these seemingly basic skills. They have difficulty interpreting their emotions and social well-being. In fact, research has shown that adolescents with AS are not reliable reporters of personal stress, anxiety, or depression. This is not because they are avoiding an uncomfortable situation or misleading themselves or others, but rather because that they often can not tell when they are feeling these emotions (Barnhill et al., 2000). Therefore, it is important to provide them with strategies that will help them understand their emotions and react in an appropriate manner to them.

Buron and Curtis (2003) created the *Incredible 5-Point Scale* to help individuals with AS understand themselves. The scale is unique in that it can be used as an obsessional index, a stress scale, a meltdown monitor, etc. Children and youth with AS are taught to recognize the stages of

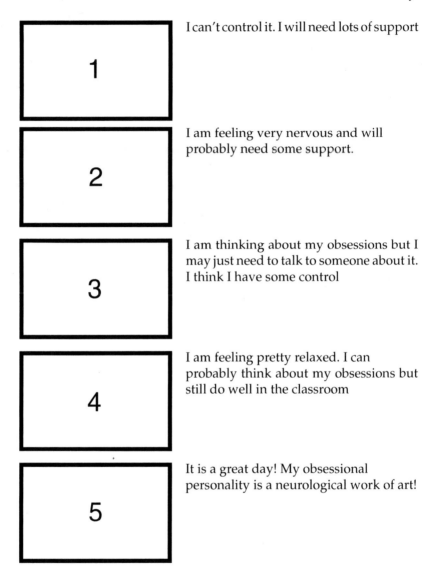

I can't control it. I will need lots of support

I am feeling very nervous and will probably need some support.

I am thinking about my obsessions but I may just need to talk to someone about it. I think I have some control

I am feeling pretty relaxed. I can probably think about my obsessions but still do well in the classroom

It is a great day! My obsessional personality is a neurological work of art!

Figure 5. Obsessional index. (*Source:* K. D. Buron, & M. Curtis (2003). *The incredible five point scale.* Shawnee Mission, KS: Autism Asperger Publishing Company)

their specific behavioral challenges and methods to self-calm at each level. Figures 5 and 6 provide two illustrations of how the *Incredible 5-Point Scale* can be used. Faherty (2000) also created a workbook for children and youth with AS to help them learn about themselves. This workbook facilitates

5 – I could lose control
4 – Can really upset me
3 – Makes me nervous
2 – Bugs me
1 – Never bothers me

Figure 6. Stress scale. (*Source*: K. D. Buron, & M. Curtis (2003). *The incredible five point scale.* Shawnee Mission, KS: Autism Asperger Publishing Company)

self-awareness through a series of exercises, such as the one presented in Figure 7.

A critical part of self-understanding is self-esteem. Ives (2001) speaks to youth with AS not only about the challenges associated with AS, but about the talents and unique gifts that are an integral part of each person. Ledgin (2002) has taken a different route to helping individuals with AS develop positive self-esteem. In his book *Asperger's and Self-Esteem: Insight and Hope Through Famous Role Models,* he has identified 13 adults who seem to share some of the characteristics of AS. Among these role models are Charles Darwin, Orson Welles, Carl Sagan, Albert Einstein, and Marie Curie. His message is that although individuals with AS have challenges, there is hope for the future, "Hope of success to which they may become entitled by their work and talent. Hope of their living a fill, happy life that is everyone's entitlement. Hope of creating for us something unique and lasting, if that is the legacy they wish their special genius to represent for all eternity" (p. 40).

Coaching

The third step in social support is coaching—helping children and youth with AS use the skills they have developed during social skills instruction and interpretation. Because individuals with AS often cognitively know skills but cannot apply them, this step is essential. A coach—parent, educator, mental health professional, or older child—upon observing the child in a social situation, can unobstrusively prompt the child to use a specific skills. Being a coach of a child or adolescent with AS requires that

Everyone feels anxious sometimes. Anxious means that a person feels worried and confused. He might cry or his hands might tremble, or he might get a stomachache or a headache. Sometimes he feels like running away or hiding. Sometimes feeling anxious makes people feel angry and they might want to scream and yell. Others might get very angry and they might want to scream and yell. Others might get very, very quiet when they are anxious.

Children with autism seem to get anxious more often than other people. I will mark what is true for me.

I feel anxious when:

- There is too much happening at the same time
- Something is just not the way it's supposed to be.
- I don't want to do something different.
- There is too much noise or bright light.
- I feel sick.
- I don't understand something.
- Someone is talking too much.
- There are too many people around; I need to be alone.
- I don't know what to do.
- I can't find the words to say.
- I make a mistake.
- I want to be alone.

- Other: _____

Figure 7. Feeling anxious. (*Source*: C. Faherty (2000). *What does it mean to me? A workbook explaining self-awareness and life lessons to the child or youth with high functioning autism or Asperger's.* Arlington, TX: Future Horizons)

the individual with AS understand the delicate balance between (a) providing support via coaching when needed and (b) allowing the student to independently use skills that he has mastered). Coaching should only be provided after the coach is certain that the child needs support to use a social skill. Coaching can take several forms: (a) feeding the language, (b) conversation starters, and (c) scripts.

FEEDING THE LANGUAGE. Adults who are feeding the language (Collins, personal communication, 1999) to children with AS are verbally prompting the child toward a social activity. The prompt may or may not contain a verbatim statement that the child is to say and is inconspicuous.

That is, the adult is extremely discrete when he feeds the language. Only the child with AS knows that he is being given social help. Feeding the language may take many forms. An adult may:

- Point out another child who is alone and might want to interact socially. *"Johnny is standing over there by himself. I think that he might want someone to play with. Why don't you go over and talk to him."*
- Provide the child with a sentence or topic he can use in a social exchange. *"Ask Susan if she has seen* Men in Black II. *If she has, you can say 'What did you like about the movie.' If she says that she hasn't seen the movie, say, "What movies have you seen lately."*

Some individuals with AS have a great degree of anxiety when they attempt to enter into a conversation or other social interaction. Feeding the language provides a jump start—a verbatim sentence or phrase that the child can use.

Feeding the language might also include the use of nonverbal cues. An adult and student with AS might have a prearranged, discrete signal that cues the child to (a) change topics, (b) ask a question of a communicative partner, or (c) move away or toward someone. Signals could include touching an earlobe or clearing the throat. When selecting a signal the adult must ensure that the signal is readily noticeable to the child but not to her peers. A second consideration is the distractibility of the signal. If the child looks intently for the signal, he may not be able to engage in a conversation with a peer—in this case, the signal becomes more important than the social interaction.

CONVERSATION STARTERS.   Beginning and maintaining a conversation requires a high degree of social skills and flexibility—two areas in which children and youth with AS have challenges. Although they want to interact with peers, some adolescents with AS don't know what to talk about. A conversation starter card, the size of a business card or trading card, can be used that contains five or six different subjects that same age peers might like to discuss. Topics are generally identified by listening to the conversations of peers in school hallways, at recess, or standing in line at a movie. It is very important that conversation started cards keep pace with current interests or activities. For example, it might be a good idea for the youth with AS whose peers often talk about music to bring up the rock group, Weezer, who just released a new CD. It would, however, be "uncool" to talk about another group whose album has been out for six months and is considered old news. This information sharer recognizes that any social interaction may include the discussion of more than one subject. Conversation cards may include topics, such as movies, musical groups, television programs, what someone did over the weekend (typically only good for

Monday conversations), or fashion. Topics must be gender sensitive as boys and girls find different topics interesting (Savner & Myles, 2000).

SCRIPTS. Scripts are a structured form of coaching. They are written sentences or paragraphs or videotaped scenarios that individuals with AS can memorize and use in social situations (Kamps, Kravitz, & Ross, 2002). They memorize and practice the scripts with an adult or other peers, then use them in real life situations. This type of coaching is used for children with AS who have difficulty generating novel language when under stress, but have excellent rote memories. Care should be taken to include "child or adolescent friendly language" in scripts. That is, common jargon should be incorporated as well as the informal language style evidenced by peers. Scripts do not work in every situation as they may make a child or adolescent sound over-rehearsed or robotic. This method is best used with model peers who understand the child, her characteristics, and the purpose of scripts.

Directions for Future Research and Practice

Little is known about the effectiveness of social skills supports for children and youth with AS. What is known, however, is that solely teaching rote skills will probably not lead persons with AS to interact successfully with others across environments. Rather, they must (a) be provided with a foundation of skills that are practical and flexible, (b) learn to understand themselves, (c) gain the skills necessary to interpret events in their environment, (c) master problem solving and conflict resolution skills, and (d) learn to generalize what they have learned to other people and situations. A cognitive approach, embedded in each of the three-tiers of social supports discussed in this chapter (instruction, interpretation, and coaching), is one that can help individuals with AS reach these goals. Behavioral techniques (i.e., time out, cognitive scripts) designed only to reduce inappropriate behaviors and teach rote social skills are not likely to meet the needs of those with AS. Children and youth with AS need to understand specific social skills as well as when, where, why, and how they are to be used. Additional research is needed to identify which cognitive-based techniques are most appropriate for specific youth and specific situations, types of generalization supports needed to ensure that children and youth with AS can use the skills they have learned, and the level of adult direction required for child success. Table 4 outlines additional issues for future consideration.

Table 4. Issues for Future Consideration and Research

- Identification of skill hierarchies in social skills
- Assessment of social skills across multiple environments
- The impact of negative role models in social skills instruction
- Assessment of vicarious learning—when and how it occurs
- Determination of how technology can be used to assess social skills
- Parents' role in selecting social targets and priorities and providing social support
- Optimal peer group composition for social skills acquisition
- The role of neurotypical peers as models in social skills groups
- How to establish criteria for mastery of social skills
- Determination of the best match of type of social support needed (i.e., intervention, interpretation, coaching) to teach specific social skills

Summary

The social needs of children and youth with AS are complex, so the interventions required to teach these skills must allow persons with AS to (a) participate in interactions that occur in complex social environments; (b) use skills in a flexible manner; (c) understand self, others, and situations that require nonliteral interpretation; and (d) be confident about themselves and their skills. A social program that includes instruction, interpretation, and coaching can help a child or adolescent with AS meet those goals.

References

Arwood, E., & Brown, M. M. (1999). *A guide to cartooning and flowcharting: See the ideas.* Portland, OR: Apricot.

Ayres, A. J. (1979). *Sensory integration and the child.* Los Angeles: Western Psychological Services.

Barnhill, G. P., Cook, K. T., Tebbenkamp, K., & Myles, B. S. (2002). The effectiveness of social skills intervention targeting nonverbal communication for adolescents with Asperger Syndrome and related pervasive developmental delays. *Focus on Autism and Other Developmental Disabilities, 17*(2), 112–118.

Barnhill, G. P., Hagiwara, R., Myles, B. S., Simpson, R. L., Brick, M. L., & Griswold, D. E. (2000). Parent, teacher, and self-report of problem and adaptive behaviors in children and adolescents with Asperger Syndrome, *Diagnostique, 25*(2), 147–167.

Baron-Cohen, S., O'Riordan, M., Stone, V., Jones, R., & Plaisted, K. (1999). Recognition of faux pas by normally developing children and children with Asperger Syndrome or high-functioning autism. *Journal of Autism and Developmental Disorders, 29,* 407–418.

Ben-Arieh, J., Myles, B. S., & Carlson, J. K. (in press). The use of a cognitive behavior modification strategy to increase on-task behavior in a student with Asperger Syndrome. *Journal of the Association of Special Education.*

Bieber J. (1994). *Learning disabilities and social skills with Richard LaVoie: Last one picked...first one picked on.* Washington, DC: Public Broadcasting Service.

Bledsoe, R., Myles, B. S., & Simpson, R. L. (2003). Use of a social story intervention to improve mealtime skills of an adolescent with Asperger Syndrome. *Autism, 7,* 289–295.

Bock, M. A. (2001). SODA strategy: Enhancing the social interaction skills of youngsters with Asperger Syndrome. *Intervention in School and Clinic, 36,* 272–278.

Bock, M. A. (2002, April 30). The impact of social behavioral learning strategy training on the social interaction skills of eight students with Asperger Syndrome. YAI National Institute for People with Disabilities 23rd International Conference on MR/DD, New York, NY.

Buron, K. D., & Curtis, M. (2003). *The incredible 5-point scale.* Shawnee Mission, KS: Autism Asperger Publishing Company.

Church, C., Alisanski, S., & Amanullah, S. (2000). The social, behavioral, and academic experiences of children with Asperger Syndrome. *Focus on Autism and Other Developmental Disabilities, 15*(1), 12–20.

Dunn, W. (1999). *The Sensory Profile: A contextual measure of children's responses to sensory experiences in daily life.* San Antonio, TX: The Psychological Corporation.

Dunn, W., Myles, B. S., & Orr, S. (2002). Sensory processing issues associated with Asperger Syndrome: A preliminary investigation. *The American Journal of Occupational Therapy, 56*(1), 97–102.

Faherty C. (2000). *What does it mean to me? A workbook explaining self-awareness and life lessons to the child or youth with high functioning autism or Asperger's.* Arlington, TX: Future Horizons.

Gagnon, E. (2001). *The Power Card strategy: Using special interests to motivate children and youth with Asperger Syndrome and autism.* Shawnee Mission, KS: Autism Asperger Publishing Company.

Goldstein, A. P., & McGinnis, E. (1997). *Skillstreaming the adolescent: New strategies and perspectives for teaching prosocial skills.* Champaign, IL; Research Press.

Gray, C. (1995). *Social stories unlimited: Social stories and comic strip conversations.* Jenison, MI: Jenison Public Schools.

Gray, C. (2000). *Writing social stories with Carol Gray.* Arlington, TX: Future Horizons.

Gray, C. A., & Garand, J. D. (1993). Social stories: Improving responses of students with autism with accurate social information. *Focus on Autistic Behavior, 8,* 1–10.

Hagiwara, T., & Myles, B. S. (1999). A multimedia social story intervention: Teaching skills to children with autism. *Focus on Autism and Other Developmental Disabilities, 14,* 82–95.

Hare, D. J. (1997). The use of cognitive-behavioural therapy with people with Asperger Syndrome. *Autism, 1,* 215–226.

Henry Occupational Therapy Services, Inc. (1998). *Tool chest: For teachers, parents, and students.* Youngstown, AZ: Authors.

Howlin, P., Baron-Cohen, S., & Hadwin, J. (1999). *Teaching children with autism to mind-read: A practical guide.* West Sussex, UK: John Wiley & Sons.

Howlin, P., & Yates, P. (1999). The potential effectiveness of social skills groups for adults with autism. *Autism, 3,* 299–308.

Ives, M. (2001). *What is Asperger Syndrome, and how will it affect me? A guide for young people.* Shawnee Mission, KS: Autism Asperger Publishing Company.

Kamps, D. M., Kravits, T., & Ross, M. (2002). Social-communicative strategies for school-age children. In H. Goldstein, L. A. Kaczmarek, & K. M. English (Eds.), *Promoting social communication: Children with developmental disabilities from birth to adolescence* (pp. 239–277). Baltimore, MD: Paul H. Brookes.

Keys, P., Trautman, M., & Mehaffey, K. (in press). *Asperger Syndrome and getting along: A conflict resolution program*. Shawnee Mission, KS: Autism Asperger Publishing Company.

Klin, A., Volkmar, F. R., & Sparrow, S. S. (2000). *Asperger Syndrome*. New York: Guilford.

Kuttler, S., Myles, B. S., & Carlson, J. K. (1998). The use of social stories to reduce precursors of tantrum behavior in a student with autism. *Focus on Autism and Other Developmental Disabilities, 13*, 176–182.

Ledgin, N. (2002). *Asperger's and self-esteem: Insight and hope through famous role models*. Arlington, TX: Future Horizons.

Lewis, T. J., Scott, T. M., & Sugai, G. (1994). The problem behavior questionnaire: A teacher-based instrument to develop functional hypotheses of problem behavior in general education settings. *Diagnostique, 19*, 103–115.

Marriage, K. J, Gordon, V., & Brand, L. (1995). A social skills group for boys with Asperger's syndrome. *Australian and New Zealand Journal of Psychiatry, 29*, 58–62.

MacLeod, A. (1999). The Birmingham community support scheme for adults with Asperger Syndrome. *Autism, 3*, 177–192.

Myles, B. S., & Adreon, D. (2001). *Asperger Syndrome and adolescence: Practical solutions for school success*. Shawnee Mission, KS: Autism Asperger Publishing Company.

Myles, B. S., Cook, K. T., Miller, N. E., Rinner, L., & Robbins, L. (2000). *Asperger syndrome and sensory issues: Practical solutions for making sense of the world*. Shawnee Mission, KS: Autism Asperger Publishing Company.

Myles, B. S., Keeling, K., & Van Horn, C. (2001). Studies using the Power Card strategy. In E. Gagnon (Ed.), *The Power Card strategy: Using special interests to motivate children and youth with Asperger Syndrome and autism* (pp. 51–57). Shawnee Mission, KS: Autism Asperger Publishing Company.

Myles, B. S., & Simpson, R. L. (2003). *Asperger Syndrome: A guide for educators and parents* (2nd ed.). Austin, TX: Pro-Ed.

Myles, B. S., & Simpson, R. L. (2001). Understanding the hidden curriculum: An essential social skill for children and youth with Asperger Syndrome. *Intervention in School and Clinic, 36*(5), 279–286.

Myles, B. S., & Simpson, R. L. (2002). Students with Asperger Syndrome: Implications for counselors. *Counseling and Human Development, 34*(7), 1–14.

Myles, B. S., & Southwick, J. (1999). *Asperger Syndrome and difficult moments: Practical solutions for tantrums, rage, and meltdowns*. Shawnee Mission, KS: Autism Asperger Publishing Company.

Parsons, S., & Mitchell, P. (1999). What children with autism understand about thoughts and thought bubbles. *Autism, 3*, 17–38.

Rogers, M. F., & Myles, B. S. (2001). Using social stories and comic strip conversations to interpret social situations for an adolescent with Asperger Syndrome. *Intervention in School and Clinic, 36*(5), 310–313.

Roosa, J. B. (1995). *Men on the move: Competence and cooperation: Conflict resolution and beyond*. Kansas City, MO: Author.

Savner, J. L., & Myles, B. S. (2000). *Making visual supports work in the home and community: Strategies for individuals with autism and Asperger Syndrome*. Shawnee Mission, KS: Autism Asperger Publishing Company.

Swaggart, B. L., Gagnon, E., Bock, S. J., Quinn, C., Myles, B. S., & Simpson, R. L. (1995). Using social stories to teach social and behavioral skills to children with autism. *Focus on Autistic Behavior, 10*, 1–16.

Szatmari, P. (1991). Asperger's Syndrome: Diagnosis, treatment, and outcome. *Pediatric Clinics of North America, 14*(1), 81–92.

Williams, K. (2001). Understanding the student with Asperger Syndrome: Guidelines for teachers. *Intervention in School and Clinic, 36,* 287–292.

Yack, E., Sutton, S., & Aquilla P. (1998). *Building bridges through sensory integration.* Weston, Ontario: Authors.

Chapter 3

Evidence-Based Instruction for Children with Asperger Syndrome

Raymond W. DuCharme

The purpose of this chapter is to identify valid and reliable approaches to the instruction of students who have an Asperger Syndrome (AS) diagnosis. A review of the research on AS on the Eric and PsychInfo databases produced 385 articles and studies for the keyword "Asperger."

The studies were then organized in a matrix for the purpose of determining which research met criteria for inclusion in the chapter. Those sources that defined diagnostic criteria of AS (*Diagnostic and Statistical Manual of Mental Disorders*, Fourth Edition [PSM-IV] or *International Classification of Diseases and Related Health Problems* [ICD-10]) and specified subject selection criteria such as age, sex, intelligence, and use of standardized measurements were included. Preference was also given to studies that described subject samples of a size over thirty and used comparison or control groups.

A clear description of experimental design and setting are important criteria for selected studies. Evidence-based approaches require sound experimental design. Evidence-based instruction and treatment are preferred to approaches based on informal data, such as interviews, single classroom observations, and case studies without controlled experimental design. Any judgment about the efficacy of a particular method of instruction must be based on evidence. To this evidence was added the 24 years of experience we have had at The Learning Clinic (TLC) working with AS youth. Relying on a social learning program model that gathers extensive ongoing data on every child enrolled in the program. We have a wealth of information that enables us to comment on educational practices for this population.

Today more children are identified as having AS, and more articles are written, but paradoxically, there is no proportional increase in valid, reliable research. Nevertheless, general information based on anecdotes and less rigorous clinical observation is influencing education practice. Review of 385 studies of AS students found forty-nine sources specific to academic instruction. Of the forty-nine articles only six used a sample size of over thirty subjects. Of the six studies that reported a sample size over thirty, some included subgroups such as ten Asperger persons, ten ADHD persons, and ten non-clinical persons as comparison groups. The total sample is over thirty, but the target group of AS students is represented by only ten subjects. All forty-nine studies reflected research design that compromised the validity and reliability of the reported outcomes.

It is surprising to discover that the research of the last dozen years provides so little empirical data on AS. However, there is a body of evidence that is helpful to the teacher and may be of heuristic value. This chapter will discuss that evidence using a pragmatic approach to both empirical and anecdotal information. Where the evidence has limitations, we note the weaknesses.

The current status of theory and research about AS requires that the teacher and clinical team develop data for each child, one child at a time, within observable pragmatic methodologies. It is the responsibility of the educator to use methods of instruction and observation to develop competencies for each student. The information in this chapter will assist the instructional team members to develop procedures that will yield data to assess the benefit to the student during his time at school.

To develop competencies the teacher will first, look at the child, examine expectations, modify the instruction, and then will assess the benefit. A pragmatic approach is described below.

- *First*, a description of the person with an AS diagnosis provides a summary of characteristics that compare similarities and differences between AS and other diagnoses.
- *Second*, the expectations inherent in the student role in a classroom are compared to the characteristics of a person diagnosed with AS.
- *Third*, the optimal program modifications for increasing classroom performance and academic success are described. Specific modifications are provided to guide academic decisions made on behalf of the person with AS.
- *Fourth*, a plan is outlined for the purpose of assessing educational benefit.

Chapter .
agnostic issues
decade. This cha
understand the st.

AS was first in
1994 (American Psyc
zation also describes .
1992). The two classific.

Dr. Hans Asperger h.   _pecific, atypical characteris..
in child behavior that he ob.   .. in the special education clinic he directed
in 1944. He and Dr. Leon Kanner were medically trained in Vienna at about
the same time. Dr. Kanner made observations of children whom he later
diagnosed with "infantile autism." Asperger's "autistic psychopathy" and
Kanner's "infantile autism" describe similar and overlapping symptoms.

Wing and Gould (1979) and Wing (1988) reported three separate dimensions to the behaviors associated with AS. Wing later added a fourth
dimension. These included (1) aloofness, (2) passivity, (3) active, odd, inappropriate approaches to others, and (4) failure to acquire social rules
through the course of normal development. While social rules may be
learned, rules are applied rigidly by the AS person.

More recent research shows an Autism Spectrum of disorders (Baron-
Cohen et al. 2001), but the defining criteria that differentiate sub-groups
are not clear. As a result, many individuals are diagnosed incorrectly. AS,
High Functioning Autism, Autism, and Non-Verbal Learning Disability
are described to have overlapping symptoms that differ in degree (Mayes
et al. 2001). These diagnostic groups as well as Schizophrenia require
more research to specify firm differentiating characteristics. Clear diagnostic categories are needed to explain etiology, academic performance, and
social development. However, the medical model of classification used
by the DSM-IV and ICD-10 may be ineffective. The degree of severity of
characteristics may best be described as points on a continuum of symptoms (Klin et al. 1995) rather than as a single diagnostic classification of
symptoms.

One such characteristic is intelligence. Educators and clinicians are
often asked to interpret the meaning of intelligence in the context of a Non-
Verbal Learning Disability diagnosis, or an AS student profile, or a child
described as High-Functioning Autistic. The current state of knowledge
provides little clear guidance to professionals who are required to provide
answers.

Intelligence

Intelligence test scores do not necessarily predict classroom success, nor do the scores predict skills associated with higher order cognitive tasks. Information processing, retention of higher order tasks, and problem solving strategies are idiosyncratic and different for each AS student. Intelligence is one factor and, often, an important asset. However, the level of cognitive inflexibility observed in the behavior of AS, HFA and NVLD students competes with the adaptability required to solve novel problems in unfamiliar problems in novel situations. Intelligence measures of normal to gifted cognitive ability are not a reliable predictor of executive function and adaptability (Rinehart, et al. 2002) among students with AS, HFA, or NVLD.

Rourke (1995), Klin et al. (1995), and Schopler et al. (1998) state that normal and higher intelligence quotients are more frequently reported for students with an AS diagnosis. AS students demonstrate, but not to a statistically significant degree, higher verbal intelligence than performance scores by about two standard deviations on WISC III test (Minshew et al. 2002). Intelligence scores indicate greater learning potential for AS students than for students with autism diagnoses who may score in the seventy-point full-scale range. The WISC-R or Stanford Binet IQ score is a helpful guide to teachers in planning instructional programs since intelligence scores are typically stable and reliable overtime (Canivez & Watkins, 1998). But even higher intelligence test scores require further analysis. The full scale score places students on the normal curve in relation to others of their chronological age. The detail in the subtest score pattern on each of the two types of tests, verbal or performance, provides a profile of specific strengths and weaknesses (Ozonoff et al. 2000).

Memory, "Anxiety," Performance

Other dimensions of AS are memory, information processing, and "anxiety," as well as the four dimensions reported by Wing and Gould (1979) and Wing (1988). All dimensions of AS may compete with learning and are associated with academic performance deficits. These same factors may be similarly present in the variations in performance of students with Autism, HFA, and NVLD. Aloofness, passivity, active odd inappropriate approaches to others, and the inability to acquire social rules through typical developmental experience may impede the AS student.

Dr. Liza Little (2001) reports that AS students experience ridicule and peer "shunning" in 94% of the cases in a survey of over 400 parent reports. Peer rejection may contribute significantly to school avoidance and to declines in academic performance. If the child avoids attending school, he is less likely to learn. Certainly AS symptoms contribute to social isolation and to the ongoing inability to develop social and communication skills with peers. Left to his own devices, the AS student has the odds against him. Positive social contact is necessary to develop the social skills needed for effective communication with others, at home, at school, or on the job.

Communication

The research on levels of pragmatic language skills demonstrated by AS students over the last decade reveals a consistent, persistent pattern of pragmatic language deficits (DuCharme & McGrady, 2003a). AS students have more difficulty communicating with peers than with adults. And they have more difficulty communicating with peers and adults than do comparison groups.

AS is, in large measure, a communication disorder. Understanding language processes illustrates that language is the partner of memory and shapes the essential concepts for social learning, pragmatic skills, and internal control over behavior. (Koning, Magill-Evans, 2001) (Jolliffe, Baron-Cohen, 1999) Language and behavior patterns become increasingly difficult to remediate as the child moves from pre-adolescence to young adulthood. Odd behaviors such as self-talk, isolation from peers, cognitive distortion, and denial of aberrant behaviors become egosyntonic and highly resistant to treatment.

AS students often appear, at first view, to be verbally bright, facile, and effective in their communication. A more careful analysis of their language structure, cognitive flexibility, word use, and especially their ability to process connotative meaning reveals substantial deficits. (Church et al. 2000)

The AS student is often characterized by teachers as literal, concrete, inflexible, and tangential in verbal expression. These behaviors become more frequent as the child moves from elementary to middle school, junior high, and high school. The AS child is then subject to an increasing number of teachers with academic content specialties. As these teachers establish personal instructional styles, classroom routines, and grading expectations, the AS child's performance becomes more discrepant with peers. As grade level increases, the level of symbolic and abstract language used by teachers also increases. The child's immersion in such language creates a situation that accentuates the child's difficulties. (Adreon & Stella, 2001)

The AS student demonstrates uneven language skill development. (Barnhill, et al. 2000) Language levels are acquired through the curriculum at developmental stages; sounds (phonemes), word bits (morphemes), semantic skills, syntax (sentence structure), discourse (large meaningful "chunks"), and meta-linguistics (higher order thinking.) As the AS child grows older, these skills appear to be more delayed. To further complicate the child's educational life, the teacher and the curriculum require receptive language skills, reading ability, and expressive language. Teachers also demand written summaries, research reports, notes, and homework.

The central point here is not to be misled by intelligence scores. Early language fluency and topical, narrow bands of expertise are often characteristics of the AS child. Further, we need to recognize that the child's language experience may be limited by his having few social contacts and few language models. Television programs and computer games are not known for high levels of language, syntax, or meta-linguistic examples. Many children demonstrate receptive language deficits that add to poor language structure.

Neurological Development

Dr. M. Levine, in his book *A Mind at a Time* (2002), discusses the differences between neurotypical functions and neurodysfunctions in the development of children. He suggests that educators need to recognize the "hidden dysfunctions" that affect children's learning and adjustment to the social demands of their environments. Dr. Levine outlines the neurodevelopmental systems that influence attention, memory, language, motor behavior, spatial ordering, sequential ordering, higher thinking, and social judgment. Dr. Levine describes the interrelationship of these systems. Further, he discusses individual and inter-system functions as they affect performance. Using student profiles, Dr. Levine reveals strengths and weaknesses in each "system" and the implications for intersystem function. The AS student profile indicates that genetics, family, environment, temperament, and emotionality as well as peers, culture, health, and education interact with intersystem functions.

Dr. Levine's point is that in his view and experience "splitting rather than lumping" children is helpful in developing treatment and educational strategies. He suggests that "lumping" children into diagnostic categories is not sufficient. We agree that individual AS profiles are best viewed in relation to structure and tasks within the education environment.

Dr. Levine alerts the reader to the meaning of neurotypical and neuroatypical functioning in children and adolescents. He minimizes, however, the importance of accurate diagnostic differentiation, and he makes only passing reference to AS. The current literature points to cognitive and social-judgment differences along a continuum. (Klin, Volkmar, & Sparrow

2000; Jolliffe & Baron-Cohen, 1999; Neihart, 2000) Such differences are best viewed as a set of concurrent symptoms that may form an identifiable pattern.

Control of Attention

We suspect that the AS child's control of attention and ability to shift attention significantly influences classroom performance. Consistent attention is absent and varies according to academic tasks and environmental influences such as class size, type of instructional method, and response mode expectations. (DuCharme & McGrady, 2002; Jackel, 1966) Control of "intake" of information and "selection" of information is also compromised for AS children, subjecting the child to stimulus overload and behavior disinhibition.

Anxiety observed as a co-morbid condition with AS may be more appropriately described as a function of "stimulus overload." The task may demand sequential steps and simultaneous responses. Under such conditions disinhibited behavior, task avoidance, accelerated speech, increase in speech volume, and requests for clarification of task requirements may produce what we see as "anxiety." The "anxious" behavior is a function of AS, an inability to process multiple stimuli.

DuCharme and McGrady (2003b) point out that the students' control over various "mind activity" may be compromised in ways that reveal tangential thinking, free associating, and day dreaming behaviors often associated with AS. Other "mind activity" such as control of the span of focus is also significant. Short attention span is directly related to the complexity of the instructional tasks, meaning the cognitive level required to perform the task, and the time allowed to complete the task. The ability to shift attention is often lacking in AS students as they may perseverate and extend their attention beyond what is expected. (Rinehart et al. 2001) Other neurotypical functions such as the pace and quality of performance and the ability to apply self-reinforcement are often compromised for an AS student. (DuCharme & McGrady, 2002)

Atypical neurodevelopment influences memory such as short-term, active mediation, and long-term functions. Memory efficiencies are positively influenced by reliable, well-rehearsed formats that involve opportunity for over learning and systematic reapplications of previously mastered material. (DuCharme & McGrady, 2003b) The AS student's memory for discrete facts may be facilitated by practice and task organization. Comprehension, analysis, synthesis, and evaluation are significantly more problematic for the AS student. (Neihart, 2000; DuCharme, 2001)

The body of literature on AS pays little attention to medication and psychopharmacological therapies for behavioral issues. The prevalence of mood and anxiety problems among children with Autism and AS (Kim et al. 2000) are well documented (Tantam, 2000) as are other co-morbid treatable conditions. The emphasis on individual differences in child neurological function is important, but not at the expense of careful differential diagnostic work and multi-modal intervention (Ozonoff et al. 2000).

Expectations Inherent in the Student Role

There is little empirical validation for specialized approaches for children with AS. Teachers often rely on newsletters, conferences, and the Internet for information. Most books for teachers are based on sporadic behavioral observation, limited samples of students, and inadequate research design. (Safran, 2001)

The Department of Psychiatry, University of North Carolina at Chapel Hill has formed a special division: Treatment, Education of Autistic and Related Communication Handicapped Children (TEACCH). Their researchers have investigated instructional methods that link structured interventions with positive outcomes for AS students (Kunce & Mesibov, 1998). The consensus is that teachers need to follow specific guidelines (Ghaziuddin & Gernstein, 1996; Strain & Schwartz, 2001):

1. Obtain current research based knowledge about AS.
2. Use both formal and informal assessment tools appropriate for AS characteristics.
3. Create a consistent and predictable environment for AS students.
4. Provide clear instructions and precise behavioral expectations with consistent follow-through.
5. Provide daily assignments, plans, and schedules.
6. Identify students' interests for motivation.

Task Analysis

The staff at The Learning Clinic (TLC) in Brooklyn, Connecticut use a task analysis approach to instruction. Task analysis is defined as the identification of the set of behaviors and abilities needed to perform a task. The AS student's initial experience with an unfamiliar task will depend on the structure of the task and the student's ability to perform the prerequisite skills needed to complete the task.

Task analysis may be classified by type, size, and kind. Three types of task analysis are *content*, *interaction*, and *prerequisite*. A *content* task analysis requires that the teacher identify teachable components, determine relationships among components, and then sequence the instructional components of the task. In content analysis, each component represents a response or set of responses, and each component is stated clearly as a behavioral objective. The relationship among components may be:

- Superordinate (A must be learned before B)
- Coordinate (Components may be learned in any order)

Interaction analysis requires the teacher to specify the teaching procedures for each component of the task. The teacher must define the degree of practice (i.e., massed or distributed). The teacher must also describe the degree of interaction with the student, such as ways to prompt, confirm, or model students' responses. The teacher's method of presenting the task must be stated. The teacher might prescribe forward chaining, backward chaining, or total task presentation.

- In forward chaining you present the elements of the task in the order that is needed to complete the task.
- In backward chaining you begin with the final product and work back to identify elements and their relationship to one another.
- In total task presentation you present the complete task along with all its elements.

The teacher prescribes the emphasis on elements and the effective presentation to match the AS students' interests.

The third type of analysis is *prerequisite* task analysis. This type of analysis defines the abilities and previous experiences needed to perform the components of the task. If the AS student is weak in prerequisite ability, the teacher may

- Teach the prerequisite skill before beginning the task.
- Adjust the material to compensate for a student weakness (e.g., dysgraphia, compensated for by use of the computer).

The *size* of the task refers to the number of units or to a skill hierarchy. The *kind* of task might be perceptual-motor as in catching a ball or buttoning a shirt. Another kind of task is *symbolic*—conceptual as in reading, writing, and computing. The more abstract the final objective, the more complex the task. Bloom's (1956) taxonomy of the cognitive domain offers examples of kinds of tasks.

The purpose of task analysis is to examine the requirements of the classroom and, more precisely, the teacher's expectations of the AS student.

Teachers often act on expectations for prerequisite behaviors that the AS student has not yet learned. When prerequisite behaviors are not clarified or taught, the AS student is likely to fail.

Content Task Analysis

The student's behavior can be examined using content analysis of teachable coordinate components. Fourteen components of behavior are described below.

1. ATTENDING BEHAVIORS. The teacher expects the student to demonstrate the following abilities:

 a. Sit in a chair at a desk for a specified period of time.
 b. Follow teacher directions.
 c. Orient to the task.
 d. Scan information from printed text.
 e. Discern task expectations from material presented.
 f. Demonstrate necessary visual-spatial capabilities.
 g. Focus attention on relevant stimuli.
 h. Control attention to apprehend and start the task.
 i. Shift attention to the appropriate task.
 j. Repeat the task.
 k. Ignore irrelevant, tangential stimuli and attend to relevant stimuli.
 l. Perform multitask operations relevant to completing the task.

The AS student is subject to distraction from sound (Bettison, 1996) and from sight. (Burack, 1994) An unfamiliar task or a task that requires an association between a previously taught concept and new application of skill will shorten task perseverance (Minshew, et al. 2002) and increase error rates (DuCharme & McGrady, 2002b).

One-to-one or small teacher-pupil ratios help the student to sustain attention. (Fondacaro, 2001) Conversely large classrooms with high student-to-teacher ratios may lead to inattention.

2. RESPONDING BEHAVIORS. The teacher in a grade level or special education classroom expects specific levels of responding behaviors such as

 a. verbal skill sufficient to communicate answers to teacher's questions or to articulate an academic-content based question or a reliable statement of feeling.
 b. pragmatic language skill at a sufficient level to comprehend communication based on social judgment that is typical for peer and adult interaction in the classroom.

c. visual motor skill prerequisite for response to the typical task format, instructional method, or assistive technology.

d. writing skills prerequisite to basic task format, and academic level required for classroom performance.

e. adequate level of comprehension of written or verbal material that requires a student response.

f. organizational, executive function skill to negotiate the classroom environment, academic task demands, homework, and/or independent organization of classroom-related materials such as teacher hand-outs, notes, note taking.

g. reading skill and reading comprehension ability required by text, CAI, or other instructional materials.

h. the ability to reliably demonstrate a level of perseverance required by the typical classroom assignment given as class work or as homework.

i. the ability to sequence information at different levels of cognitive complexity so as to meet the academic task requirement of the instructional material.

j. Memory skills.
   1. Short-term memory
   2. Long-term memory
   3. Memory for facts
   4. Associative memory
   5. Memory for denotative and annotative items

The ability to demonstrate sufficient memory skills to acquire and retain academic content is often assumed. The student is expected to recall and apply the strategies and content when elicited by task requirements. All of these skills are part of the expectations inherent in the student role.

The behaviors described as responding present problems for the student who shows the characteristics of AS. Verbal skills are present within a narrow band of interest, but broad based knowledge and skill are typically absent. Problem-solving, facile recall of past solutions, and verbal negotiation are also absent skills. The TLC Pragmatic Language Skill Survey indicates consistent and persistent deficits in four categories of communication; topic, purpose, abstraction, use of visual-gestural cues (DuCharme, R. & McGrady, K. 2003a). Organization skills, inferential comprehension, memory, perseverance, sequencing, and ordering part-whole relationships are reported to be problems for AS students.

3. REINFORCEMENT BEHAVIORS.   This pertains to a student's ability to

a. provide contingent positive social reinforcement appropriate to setting, situation, and persons (peer or adult).

b. assert negative reinforcement in a contingent and appropriate way.

    c. receive, process, and respond appropriately to positive reinforcement and other classroom incentives such as grades, awards, status.

    d. perceive, accept, and understand negative reinforcement offered by authorities, peers, adults, and other persons.

    e. demonstrate a level of motivation in response to either positive or negative reinforcement used in the classroom setting.

    f. demonstrate evidence of a hierarchy of internal self-reinforcement consistent with classroom values and sanctions.

    g. create hierarchical menu of positive reinforcers.

    h. show a positive response to vicarious reinforcement used in the classroom such as imitation of student behavior following the positive reinforcement of that student's behavior.

The student's underreaction to reinforcing stimuli is observed in relation to motivation. Reinforcement is observed as a cue to associate behavior and responses rather than as a motivator for future performance. Sustained, goal oriented behavior is absent, thereby making delayed reinforcement ineffective. Little reinforcement, positive or negative, is offered by the students at TLC in their spontaneous interactions with others.

Punishment, on the other hand, through response cost systems, loss of activity, status, or privilege is observed to elicit anger, threat, avoidance, and defiant behavior.

4. INITIATING BEHAVIORS. Task initiation includes the following abilities:

    a. direct oneself so as to anticipate and comply with classroom routines

    b. follow directions provided by computer assisted instructions

    c. follow teachers' directions to begin classroom tasks, activities, transitions

    d. start a task according to directions in the text

    e. begin tasks that require the student to use visual-graphic-icon cues

It is observed that self-direction, teacher-direction, and written direction are unreliable methods to elicit task initiation. Computer assisted rehearsal, teacher-coached performance, and the use of icons and visual-graphic directions are effective. These conclusions are based on single subject, multiple baseline, repeated measure designs assessed over time at TLC.

5. COMPLYING BEHAVIORS. This refers to the student's ability to meet task criteria and teacher standards. Task compliance is shown by

    a. accepting correction from teachers, aides, and sometimes peers

    b. accepting correction in the public, open situation of the classroom

c. correcting assignments, reading assignments, redoing assignments in a way that corresponds to a predetermined standard

These behaviors—attending, responding, reinforcement, initiating, and complying with standards—present major obstacles to a student with a diagnosis of AS. The ability to meet task criteria and teacher standards is dependent upon the fit between the student, the task, and task analysis. If the task analysis is correct, and a mastery learning model is used that allows the student to repeat trials and to correct errors, then standards are predictably met (DuCharme, 2001). Teacher-centered instructional methods, lecture formats, and delayed correction and feedback to students are not effective, as measured by student performance on academic tasks.

Additional expectations that may reveal problems for the AS student are examined below.

6. COMPLETING BEHAVIORS. The ability of the student to finish the assignment depends on

a. performing specific tasks according to the presented method
b. working independently
c. returning a completed product to the teacher

7. TRANSITIONING BEHAVIORS. The ability to move from one task to the next and to recognize when to stop one task and begin another depends on

a. taking independent steps between tasks (e.g., the student can follow a multi-step strategy to solve a math problem and then change from math to science or other kind of task)
b. recognizing and using prompts that signal the need to move from one task to another

8. COOPERATING BEHAVIORS. Students are expected to display and maintain a demeanor appropriate to the classroom such as

a. taking turns in discussion
b. waiting for another person to finish speaking
c. avoiding arguing
d. maintaining appropriate speech volume
e. sharing equipment (e.g., computer time)
f. avoiding ridicule of peers
g. displaying appropriate posture
h. maintaining eye contact
i. requesting to exit the classroom

AS students, though desiring positive peer relationships, are ill equipped to control their odd behaviors, clinical symptoms, and poor pragmatic language deficits. Soderstrom (et al. 2002) report on characteristics of adults with an AS diagnosis. The most common (AS) temperament is characterized by obsessive, passive dependent and explosive features. The AS individual demonstrates a desire for peer relationship and attempts to fit into mainstream expectations (Jones & Meldal, 2001). Little (2001) conducted a peer-victimization survey with a response rate of four hundred and forty-one (70%) parents of AS and NVLD students. The survey data is arranged by age, gender, and diagnosis. Ninety-four percent of the respondents reported assault or shunning by peers and siblings.

9. Competing Clinical Behaviors. The classroom norm expects AS students to work without distracting or disturbing others. Ann Wagner and Kathleen McGrady (see chapter 4) discuss clinical issues associated with an AS diagnosis and review psychiatric symptoms and co-morbid conditions. The teacher must prescribe instruction that competes with the clinical symptoms listed below.

    a. perseveration on a topic not related to the classroom instruction
    b. obsessive thought
    c. inability to shift topics from personal view to data based view
    d. threatening behavior, verbal aggression
    e. dichotomous thinking—win—lose orientation to discussion
    f. confabulation
    g. affirming false (data) information
    h. not taking responsibility for own actions, resisting accountability
    i. stealing
    j. sexually inappropriate comments
    k. violation of personal boundaries
    l. cognitive disorientation, distortion of information

The combination of evidence-based instruction, medication therapy, and cognitive behavioral therapy are recommended for treatment. Behaviors such as speaking out, exiting the classroom without permission, expressing tangential ideas, self-talk, or other behaviors may be reduced (DuCharme & McGrady, 2003b).

10. Adapting Behaviors. The ability to move from class to class, and to follow the teacher's prescribed schedule requires explicit directions. Different teachers may have different classroom procedures and schedules. Some teachers have unpredictable, flexible routines that present change in each class. Such classrooms may be described as unilateral and unreliable.

To adapt to classroom routines the student must learn to

    a. identify the particular schedule and routine of each classroom
    b. follow the schedule and routine

"Closed" classroom environments, such as self-contained classrooms or schools that prescribe consistent routines, provide greater structure and predictability. The AS student will more readily learn the reliable expectations of a closed setting. Such classrooms are described as unilateral and reliable.

"Open settings" are environments that require multiple transitions within and between classrooms. The "open setting" requires that the student initiate and regulate performance and cooperation. "Open settings" are most suited for group activities that are interactive and oriented toward symbolic—conceptual tasks. The complexity of the task requires a high degree of ability to solve abstract problems. "Open settings" are the most difficult for the AS student to negotiate.

11. COOPERATING WITH MEDICATION ADMINISTRATION.   The ability of the student to accept his need for and use of medication may be prerequisite to performing in the classroom. The student's ability to accept the need for medication on a prescribed schedule may also be prerequisite. The probability that an AS student will require medication as part of a dual-diagnosis with co-morbid conditions for treatment is increasing. Attention deficit disorders, bipolar disorders, depression, and other mental health conditions require a regimen of medications. The need for prescribed medications to be taken during the school day and at times in the classroom is more evident. (Ghaziuddin et al. 1998) (Kim et al. 2000)

Important skills to teach are

    a. following prescribed schedules of medication
    b. managing one's own medication

TLC uses a specific teaching procedure to enable AS students to demonstrate reliable self-administration of medication. This skill is a prerequisite for a student's acceptance into an independent living program.

12. DEPENDING ON STRUCTURE.   It is reported in anecdotal and clinical observations that students with an AS diagnosis are structure dependent. The researches at TLC over the past decade support such observations. The general school curricula includes recess, physical education, music, art, and lunch visits as part of a weekly student schedule. These types of activities are less structured, more open, more dependent on self-initiation and self-regulation. Most AS students have problems with less structured activities.

Art and music are particularly important experiences for AS students since these activities often coincide with abilities and interests. The structure of the activity, task type, size, and kind are related to the student's successes. In physical education classes the student's gross motor awkwardness may compete with success or participation.

Recess and cafeteria time are most problematic for AS students. At these times the student's social oddity, poor pragmatic language, self-talk, and fast walking offer targets for peer ridicule and shunning.

13. COMPLETING HOMEWORK. The completion of homework to fulfill standards and submission of work on time are two of the most frequent complaints of parents and students about teacher requirements. The lack of homework preparation and failure to complete the work on time result in poor grades and discipline issues. Independent work at home and study time at school require that students remember academic strategies and apply them appropriately. The student is also expected to be sufficiently organized to remember books and materials needed for independent work.

14. ATTENDING SCHOOL. The ability to maintain regular attendance at school is a critical component of classroom performance. Mastery of patterns and expectations are associated with regular attendance. All of the above components of performance expectations are factors in a student's attendance or avoidance of school and the classroom.

Regular school attendance doesn't always predict classroom attendance. A recently referred student to TLC produced a record of excellent school attendance. The vice-principal was his "best friend" as he spent most of his school day in the principal's office and not in his classroom.

Our content analysis of classroom expectations is not all inclusive, nor have we presented teachable subcomponent skills hierarchies. However, the list of tasks do present a picture of misfit between the characteristics of AS and the expectations inherent in a classroom.

Cognitive Resources

Cognitive Load Theory (CLT) offers research that is particularly relevant to precise task analysis of academic content. CLT is concerned with the manner in which cognitive resources are focused and used during learning and problem solving (Sweller & Chandler, 1991). The main goal is to guide decisions about instructional design. A complete discussion of CLT is provided in special issue of *Educational Psychologist* (2003).

CLT explores the relationship between instructional task design and the academic performance of AS students.

CLT is based on assumptions about human cognitive structure. The theory postulates the relationships between long term memory capacity, schema of mental representation of knowledge, and limited processing capacity of working memory. The mechanisms of working memory have executive control over visual-spatial information such as text and pictures and the phonological loop for spoken text or music. Understanding the limits of capacity and independence of function of these systems may shed light on mastery issues associated with AS.

Measuring cognitive load depends upon self-report measures and objective measures such as physiological, behavioral, and learning outcome measures. The measurement of cognitive load as part of task design and analysis helps us to define the difficulty of different types of learning materials. Learned information may be recalled and applied by AS students according to its cognitive load measures.

Toward an Optimal Classroom

The recommended instructional methods were tested at TLC with students diagnosed with AS according to DSM-IV criteria, male and female in a ratio of eight-to-one, of adolescent age, and demonstrating a dual diagnosis that includes attention deficit disorder, depression, anxiety disorder, specific learning disability, obsessive compulsive disorder, and aggressive patterns of behavior. All the students demonstrated normal to gifted intelligence quotients as measured by the WISC-R III.
During a ten-year period one hundred and fifty Asperger students, were referred for services because of school failure, school avoidance, and clinical issues. All the students were identified through the IDEA procedures and standards in order to be eligible for special services and meet section 504 criteria.

The following list of instructional modifications for the student with an AS diagnosis are outlined by topic and key factors. An "optimal" modification is stated as a general recommendation. For example, if *identification of staff* is the topic and key factors are listed as:

- number of staff interacting with each student
  - each period
  - each morning
  - each afternoon
  - total individual staff each day
- definition of staff role
  - primary staff—self-contained classroom
  - content specialist teacher

- ○ teacher—disciplinarian
- ○ academic teacher and social skill teacher and counselor
- ○ teacher—subject—tutor

then the recommendation is:

> *Optimal.* Optimal is defined to be the staff role that will yield the greatest benefit to the student. The optimal staff role in the example above prescribes one "coach" for monitoring student performance and providing academic tutorial and social skill instruction in-vivo; all classes.

Instructional Setting

The "open" versus "closed" environmental influence on social learning and compliant behavior is described by Tharpe & Wetzel (1969) in their examination of the variables connected to behavior modification in the natural environment. Open environments require self-regulation of transitions, interactions with others, and movement in space. "Closed" environments provide external control over behavioral options, number and type of transitions, pre-planned schedules, social and instruction prompts, and degrees of personal freedom earned through reinforcement menus based on standards for performance.

> *Optimal.* Behavioral standards and choices designed for AS students are limited, precise, and based on the level of self-regulation ability. A closed environment is more effective for instruction and social skill development than an open environment.

Class Size

Adolescent students in TLC programs report that the size of the group is important to them. The instructional task and level of complexity also influences their ability to master new academic information. There appears to be, according to student reports, a relationship between the task, the size of the instructional group, and the rate of learning (DuCharme & McGrady, 2002).

> *Optimal.* Teachers' experience over the past twenty years shows that the optimal group size is over three students but under ten. One-on-one instruction, in tutorial format is best to introduce new, complex cognitive material and to monitor the acquisition rate and retention of skills.

Environmental Structure

According to *Webster's New International Dictionary, Unabridged* (1934) definition, structure refers to "the interrelation of parts as dominated by the general character of the whole, as the structure of society or the structure of a sentence . . . "Structure, then, is an organization of parts in order to make a unified whole. The student with an AS diagnosis requires a cohesive, precise, educational structure. The student's success depends on the way in which the structure of the child's experience at school is defined and communicated.

A whole school approach is designed to coordinate expectations, standards of conduct, sanctions, and student-staff roles across settings. This appears most beneficial when designed on the basis of the student's developmental needs (Grace 1998).

TLC accomplishes the aim of designing a defined structure by employing the whole school with fidelity of treatment model. An example of the effect of fidelity of treatment is shown by an orchestra. In a group of wonderfully talented musicians, one might perform a solo, the strings would have their part, and the brasses theirs. An orchestra leader conducts. The sheet music keeps everyone focused on the piece. Each musician plays particular notes. Harmony passes to our senses and we experience melody. But what happens when a musician plays an unrelated sheet of music? Discord. Discord in the experience of children with AS is a negative and serious outcome.

There are various means to communicate structure to the student. The structure may be cued by the adult staff with clear, succinct verbal messages. The environment may be arranged to prompt student behavior. A procedural education and treatment approach is used by TLC staff in the form of a written manual.

Optimal. Cues and prompts are needed to maintain the student's perception of the structure designed for him. Guided instruction is optimal for successful task completion.

- Daily plans and standards for self-monitoring their performance during and at the completion of an academic task is consistently reported as helpful by students.
- Checklists and digital devices (organizers) provide prompts and reminders that assist students in keeping schedules.
- Assigned work stations, individual computers, pre-written daily plans, and schedules for each student can serve as prompts.

- Peer-coaching or tutorial may guide student performance with text or script for additional guidance.
- Icons and ideograms illustrate steps needed to perform tasks.

Discipline

The need for a reliable system of discipline is one of the most frequent requests of students at TLC. Many students perceive rules in their previous schools as not enforced reliably. The "inflexible" approach of AS students to rules and their reliance on predictable structure contribute to their sensitivity about "rule breakers."
Students report that they want to "know the rules". They want rules to be consistently applied. They want the whole school to have the same rules, standards and sanctions.

Students with AS are frequently the "junior attorneys" of the school. They quickly recognize violations of rules in others that go unpunished. They explain how their behavior doesn't quite fit the description of a violation.

The Learning Clinic has developed and employed a behavior management flow chart that is used in all parts of the program—school, residence, and home environments (Figure 1). A written manual explains the use of the flow chart for staff, students, and parents.

The effectiveness of the flow chart is noted in the clarity of direction given to students, the time allowed to understand the direction, and the consequences. The clarity of direction states what the student is to do. The direction is precise, brief and within the response repertoire of the child. Then, at least ten seconds are given for the student to process the request and to respond. The ten-second time for response is based on researches by DuCharme in 1972 that measured response latencies for children of different development ages when given verbal learning tasks. The use of the flow chart results in consistent improvement in compliance and decreases the need for negative consequences.

The teacher's ability to wait a sufficient amount of time for a student to process a request and to respond is critical to the student's ability to comply with the request. We have observed students who had been defined as "elective mute". The "mute behavior" is indicative of the student's inability to respond within the time allowed by the teacher. The child may require more time to formulate and express a response than is allowed. In such cases, the child is not mute. He simply requires more time than the teacher typically allows him to answer.

Optimal. A precise, reliable, schoolwide behavior management system in combination with clear verbal directions and sufficient time allowed for response is best for AS students.

Student Diagnosis and Classroom Mix

The diagnoses of other students in the classroom are important. The diagnosis of AS, even with co-morbidity, is compatible with some diagnostic groups and not others. First, the co-morbidity associated with an AS diagnosis determines inclusion criteria. Analysis of the mix of AS students with students who have other disabilities raises certain questions. Is the ratio of diagnosed to non-diagnosed students discernable to the teacher? If so, is the teacher able to teach children within the range of diagnoses? Can students who have medical needs be served given the mix of clinical issues? Is the student intelligence quotient a factor for inclusion or exclusion in the class?

AS students are diagnosed within a normal to gifted intellectual range. Frequently, in our experience students with intelligence quotients of 70 or lower have an erroneous AS diagnosis. The instructional methods and curricula for a student with an IQ of 70 are profoundly different than those for students with a 136 quotient.

AS students do not perform well socially or academically in classes with students diagnosed with conduct disorders or disruptive or aggressive behaviors. The AS student is intimidated and/or exploited by students who are prone to victimize their more vulnerable peers.

Optimal. The absence of students who have below average IQ, conduct disorder, acting out—aggressive behavior is optimal for a student with an AS diagnosis in the classroom.

TEACHER-TO-STUDENT RATIO. The teacher-student ratio depends upon a number of variables such as type, size, and kind of task, number of classroom distractions, clinical issues, and level of skill that the student is able to demonstrate. The range of options for instructional ratios also depends upon school resources. The optimal group size for general instruction is over three and under ten students. But within that range, it must be noted, that the preferred ratio is one-to-one when new information, instructional strategy, or novel application is to be taught.

Optimal. One-to-one tutorial instruction is best for the AS student in the classroom.

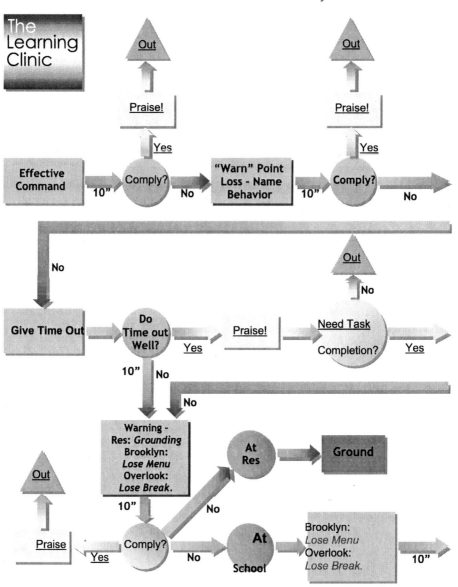

Figure 1. Behavior Management Flow Chart.

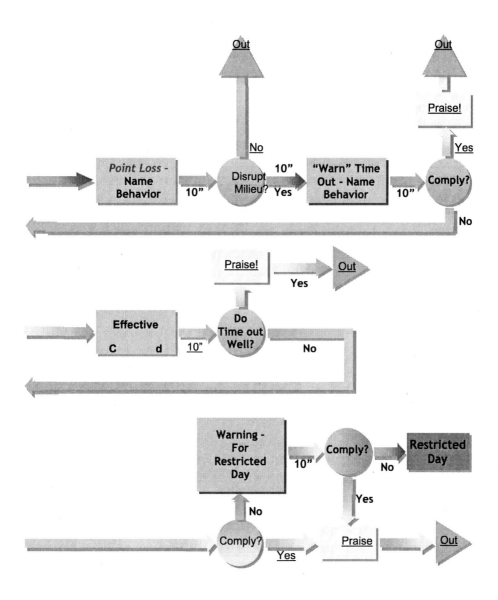

LEGEND

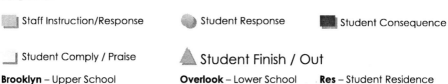

Staff Instruction/Response   Student Response   Student Consequence

Student Comply / Praise   Student Finish / Out

Brooklyn – Upper School   **Overlook** – Lower School   **Res** – Student Residence

Instructional Methods

It's informative to measure the social perceptions of AS students because they are so often wrong. Given the complexity of human relationships and the uses and misuses of language, we can expect sometimes to deceive ourselves and to misread others. But not seventy percent of the time, as is observed in the social judgments of AS students (DuCharme, & McGrady, 2003a).

Their tendency to misread social cues makes AS students particularly vulnerable to methods using collaboration. On the other hand, students can benefit from methods that are consistent, reliable, impersonal, individually paced, and interesting. Resistant learners and students who are interested and familiar with computer assisted instruction (CAI) benefit from the use of CAI.

The best methods for students with an AS diagnosis are based on the individual's characteristics. The general characteristics of AS students are also important. The significant identifying markers of AS in current literature (Klin et al. 1995, Schopler, 1998, Frith, 1991) are

1. absence of desire for social interaction and avoidance of social interaction; misperception of social cues
2. pragmatic deficits and decrease in competence with complex and abstract levels of language processing requirements; preference for picture cues and ideagrams
3. restricted, repetitive patterns of behavior
4. language processing difficulties and expressive language response latency
5. resistance to criticism and performance evaluation by teachers and others
6. sensory overload response to loud noise, too much verbal information, textual material with a "dense" level of content, unregulated pace of questioning, and short time interval in response requirement
7. negative responses to personal judgments of correct–incorrect performance
8. deficits in short-term memory and recall of previously learned material

Optimal. The methodology that competes best with the issues listed above is academic task presentation through computer assisted instruction (CAI). Such instruction provides

- consistent format
- reliable mode and pace of presentation of tasks
- progressive increases in task complexity based on performance evidence
- rapid, contingent, correct-incorrect response feedback and scoring

- controlled learning pace
- impersonal presentation and assessment
- motivation based on interests of AS students
- a controlled pace for reading text to the student

The computer-assisted tutorial format has been effective for hundreds of students over a twenty year period at TLC based on individual (single subject) performance reviewed weekly and quarterly as measured by an 80% criterion.

CAI is a flexible method that may be used in a tutorial format, in dyadic collaboration, or in small group collaboration under teacher direction. TLC staff have recorded daily performance in each type of instructional format for AS with high degree, 80% or above, successes during repeated application.

CAI methods are more effective than teacher-directed, group discussions or self-regulated learning models for AS students. The computer can correct spelling, present word choices, and assist with punctuation and organization. Further, help is cued by icons that support the AS student's preference for visual systems. CAI methods can include assistive technology such as the reader-scanner, Alternative Learning System curricula, "Co-Writer", "Inspiration" and other text—CAI coordinated materials.

Interpersonal Style

The teacher's interpersonal styles are related to the student's success in the classroom. Observations of fifty different staff-student interactions over the past twenty-years suggests that the teacher's characteristics make a difference. AS students appear to consistently benefit from teachers who are calm, clear, and positive in their communication.

"*Directness*" in communicating expectations and performance results avoids the problem of misunderstanding. "Directness" also decreases the need to revise messages, repeat directions, or correct student responses.

A *nonjudgmental* approach to student behavior is helpful. Asperger students are observed to react negatively to being told what they do wrong. The focus on "what to do" rather than "what was done wrong" is most productive. The AS student often seizes on the negative correction and perseverates. A calm, low key personal demeanor appears to have a reassuring and calming effect on student behavior. The teacher who is precise, relevant to the student's interests, organized, and consistent has fewer problems with AS students. Further, student productivity rises in non-judgmental settings.

The most effective teachers are those who focus on positive behavior and on behaviors that, if demonstrated by the student, will compete with or replace problem behaviors. Allowing negative or task-irrelevant behavior to occur is risky for both teacher and student. Learning a replacement behavior or corrective action is more difficult than practicing a correct response from the start.

Avoid correction, with an emphasis on what is incorrect or with review of the error and attention to why the answer is wrong, produces unintended outcomes and resistance to redirection.

> *Optimal.* Much better, in our experience, is a "backward" chain task analysis. Demonstrate the correct answer, solution, or sequence of steps from the desired result to the first step. Provide the student with a model of the correct answer and then teach the components.

Task Design and Academic Risk

The complexity of the task and the requirements of answering a question are variables that risk the student's success. Non-compliance and symptoms of perseveration, rigidity, oppositionality, and "anxiety" may be a response to a transition, especially if the transition is out of the ordinary routine and is not well rehearsed in advance.

> *Optimal.* Take the needed time to rehearse the student by explaining the need for a transition. State precisely how and when the transition will be made. Allow sufficient time for rehearsal prior to the transition. Maintain continuity during rehearsal, the transition, and the completion of the transition. A staff "coach" should have the role to support transitions with rehearsal.

Before presenting a question the teacher should ask: What are the parts of a multi-level question? What is the cognitive level required by the vocabulary in the question? What is the student to infer that the answer requires? The cognitive "load" of the question is important and must fit the student's level of ability (Bloom, 1964). The structure of the question, the student's pre-assessed knowledge, and exposure to evaluation and judgment are risk factors to control and to gradually increase. Response modes available to the student may add or detract from risk. If a written response is required, and a time limit is placed on the answer, the risk is increased. If the student must read an answer aloud, additional risk is present.

Too much risk will prevent a student from demonstrating skills and abilities. The lack of an answer may not signify a lack of knowledge, but rather the student's inability to answer a question with the level of risk present. The manner in which the teacher enables the student to develop a tolerance for academic risk may vary. But the principle is the same: Taking risks is a skill and can be taught.

The teacher's level of sensitivity and creativity cannot be overestimated as an influence on the student's success. To illustrate, a teacher was observed speaking quietly, almost secretly, with a student who had a distressed look on his face. He stated that a scary movie about two girls would not leave his mind. The child said that he could not do his work. The teacher took an empty plastic container that had previously held a cookie and calmly said, "When the scary thought comes into your mind, then blow it into this box and cover it with the lid." The boy blew into the box and calmly reported to his teacher that, "It works!" He was very concerned when later that morning the lid fell from the box. He scurried to replace it.

> *Optimal.* Control the level of academic risk in task design. When matching a teacher to a student with an AS diagnosis, stress the importance of an organized, calm, reliable, and creative approach.

Classroom Routine

The standard expectation at TLC is that each student, given an appropriate task and curricula, will complete twenty-six graded assignments to a minimum standard of 80% correct each academic quarter. Academic performance is self-paced and governed by the completion of designated objectives, not by time spent in class.

Each student, with the teacher's help, establishes a daily schedule of academic subjects with time allotted and specific objectives for each subject. Academic performance is assessed by the end of each day, and a plan for the next day is started.

The number of assignments to be completed each day is recorded as well as the number of assignments that are incomplete and do not meet the 80% standard criterion. Higher level cognitive material requires a higher standard of 90%. The number of assignments and number of times assignments are redone to meet criteria is also recorded. The teacher adjusts the number of assignments per subject each day to ensure a practical expectation for performance. Assignments are adjusted according to ability level.

The student is given time in the schedule to select topics and tasks of interest. Opportunity for collaborative activity with selected peers and other adults is part of the student schedule. No homework is required other than reading or independent non-graded researches based on student interest. Note taking in class is rarely a requirement.

A balance is necessary between tutorial instruction and collaborative learning. Most important is the teacher's opportunity to schedule focused dialogues with each student. Talking about their writing, music, and art are important to students who are developing a pattern to externalize their thought and to consider the responses of others.

Optimal. Schools should use *all* the strategies and procedures described above with significant effect for AS students.

Transitions

Transitions are defined as the changes in locations, attention, and responses to tasks that are required of a student.

An examination of transitions required by textbooks, workbooks, teachers' interpersonal styles, methods, and daily movements of people reveals hundreds of changes each day. If a child's symptom profile includes decreases in competencies and self-regulation during transitions, then we have probably created too many changes for the child. Programs with significant numbers and types of transitions are not easily negotiated.

Transitions in "performance" expectations on a single page of text may be too numerous for the student to handle. Attentional shifts required by changes in task demands or because of distractions, alter the AS student's performance.

The teacher is advised to assess the degree of self-regulation expected of the student in the classroom. Expectations may change from one setting to another during and after transitions. Consider expectations of self-regulation along a continuum of supervision by staff, from continuous supervision to 90% supervision, then 80%, 70%, 50%, 25%, and finally none. The behavior of the student at different locations, during different activities, and at different times with different instructional groups will provide the data needed to select optimal levels of supervision.

Students have reported difficulty during physical education classes, particularly in locker rooms. At this time when the instructor is providing "privacy", the AS student is most frequently victimized by teasing or aggression. The teacher must identify when maximum supervision is necessary.

Optimal. During transitions the teacher must provide 80–90% supervision unless the data indicates that it is not needed. The decision about the level of supervision is best made by direct staff observation during various activities at different times. Such decisions are not based solely on the student's report of incidents.

Non-compliance and symptoms of perseveration, rigidity, oppositionality, and "anxiety" may be a response to a request for a transition, especially when the transition is not well rehearsed. Teachers must take the time to rehearse the student by explaining the need for a transition and the steps to follow. Allow sufficient time prior to the transition for rehearsal, but maintain continuity in time from the rehearsal through the transition to its completion. A staff "coach" should have the role of easing transitions by necessary rehearsal.

Clinical Services

The AS student's academic performance and rate of skill acquisition may be significantly influenced by anxiety, depression, compulsion, attention deficit, and other treatable conditions.

The role of the clinical staff, school psychologist, psychiatrist, and nurse must be clarified in relation to their roles that support the instructional program. A cohesive, seamless approach is necessary in each instructional setting and during non-academic activities at school such as recess and cafeteria times.

Clinicians are important to the teacher because they provide direct services to students that help the student adjust to classroom expectations. Further, the clinician is important to the teacher as a consultant and observer. The consultant may provide data on student-to-student interaction and teacher-to-student interaction. The instructional task, method, response modes required, and response latency demonstrated by student patterns of responses contribute to a data base provided to the teacher.

Behavioral standards for the instructional setting require objective description and assessment. The design of the setting can either meet or compete with the needs of the students with AS. To illustrate, during a recent visit by this author to a hospital school, resident students demonstrated the relationship between small classrooms, student deficits, and behavioral disruptions in the classroom. Too many students with limited self-regulation ability were placed in a small classroom. The result was student-to-student aggression, assault on the teacher, and increased amount of time spent by students in restraint and/or in their living units. Conversely, examining TLC quarterly reports on aggression, need for supervision or restraint or seclusion demonstrate that a properly designed environment which provides the appropriate degree of structure eliminates occurrences of the intense behaviors that require students to leave the classroom.

Assessing Benefits to Students

An evidence-based intervention model typically collects data on each student's performance for the purpose of assessing its benefits. The data provides a stimulus for modifying services when performance measures indicate the need for changes. Continuous monitoring of each student's performance enables staff to assess the intended and unintended outcomes that result from changes of teacher, classroom, task, or medication.

In evidence-based instruction data are collected daily at specified intervals, using the interval frequency method of recording. Frequency and percentage of occurrence of selected behaviors are charted weekly and summarized in the form of quarterly reports. The data are then shared with administrators, educators, and clinical staff.

Evidence-based approaches provide opportunities to analyze the AS student's success with factors related to instruction, task organization, response formats, motivation, and feedback systems.

Examples

The Learning Clinic provides evidence-based education and treatment at two locations; the Brooklyn and Overlook Schools. Performance data is collected and reported for each site separately for comparison purposes. The types of data and the student scores are presented in data Figures 2 and 3.

Data are collected to show the number of students at each school site, the number of days available for instruction, and the total number of student absences. The percentage of absences provides telling information about the availability of students, each quarter to their instruction program. The lower the percent of absences, the better for academic and social performance. Behavioral averages report level of student compliance with school behavioral standards. The self-evaluation system is labeled "OPS", the abbreviation for "Off The Point System." OPS means that the student demonstrates sufficient self-regulation so as not to require the point-based cueing system. OPS students provide self-report data.

A manual of performance standards governs staff and students. The manual provides instructions to staff as to behavioral definitions, and observation and reliability measures. The higher the behavior average, the fewer the rule violations in evidence. Students' scores that are 80% or above meet the program standard for compliance and indicate a generally positive level of self-regulations within the program structure.

Suspensions, "restricted" days, and "stopped programs" all indicate significant lack of influence of treatments over student behavior. Such data provide a stimulus for modifying student services.

The academic scores for each student are calculated on the basis of a minimum of twenty-six graded assignments each quarter. The grades are based on a 100 point system. An 80% criterion is the program standard for mastery of each assignment.

The first quarter of the 2002/2003 school year encompassed 43 school days. Data for the quarterly report was collected from the students' 1st quarter reports. Data is reported by building.

	Brooklyn	Overlook
Number of students	25	37
Attendance		
Number of absences/available days	1075/60	1591/62
Percentage of absences	5%	3%
Behavioral Averages	92.2%	95.2%
90% or above	20 students or 80%	28 students or 76%
80%–89%	4 students or 16%	4 students or 11%
70%–79%	0 students or 0%	1 students or 2%
69% or below	0 students or 0%	0 students or 0%
OPS	1 students or 4%	1 students or 2%
N/A	0 students or 0%	3 students or 9%
Home suspensions (days)	0	0
Stopped programs (days)	0	0
Restricted days (days)	6	33
Academic Averages	91.4%	91.7%
90% or above	19 students or 76%	25 students or 68%
80%–89%	6 students or 24%	5 students or 14%
70%–79%	0 students or 0%	0 students or 0%
69% or below	0 students or 0%	0 students or 0%
N/A	0 students or 0%	7 students or 18%
Extended Day Students	21	26
Extended Day Behavior Averages	98.1%	97.8%
90% or above	20 students or 95%	24 students or 92%
80%–89%	1 students or 5%	2 students or 8%
70%–79%	0 students or 0%	0 students or 0%
60% or below	0 students or 0%	0 students or 0%
OPS	0 students or 0%	0 students or 0%
N/A	0 students or 0%	0 students or 0%

Figure 2. The Learning Clinic First Quarter Report, 2002/2003.

Performance in "extended day" is measured each day, Monday through Thursday, during activities provided after regular academic classes. Specific, individualized behavioral and social-skill objectives are operationally defined and assessed daily. Scores are recorded by staff and then through student self- assessment. The scores are based on a 100 point high—0 low scale. An 80% score is the criterion for mastery of each type of skill.

Name	Eng	Lit	Math	S.S.	Sci	Misc	Misc	Total	Avg
Elaine		90	88		94	89	90	451	90.2
Christine	91	93	90	91		95	92	552	92
Kathy				87		91		178	89
Chris	87	96	90	91	92	95		550	91.8
Ron	92	85	91		94			362	90.5
Karen	80	80	94	89	92			435	87
Joe		95	92		95			282	94
John		97	89	91	90	92	100	559	93.1
Jim				93	99			192	96
Bob	80		86	87	80			333	83.2
Bill		90	89	92	91	95		457	91.4
Mike	93	95	89	90		92	92	551	91.8
Adam		95	92	94	93	96	98	568	94.6
Len	94	90	96	94	95			469	93.8
George	92	95	90	97	91	91	90	646	92.2
Rob	95	95	91	94	97	92		564	94
Erica	91	88	95	93	86	90	88	631	90.1
Jill	88		92			89	92	350	87.5
Sally	94	95	97	99	98	95		578	96.3
Joy		92	92	92	94	91	92	553	92.1
Alan	95	95	95	97	94			476	95.2
Mike	88	99		95	95	90	94	561	93.5
Kristen	90		99		93	91		373	93.2
Steve	80	80	92	89				341	85.2
								2285.7 91.4%	

Figure 3. Brooklyn—Academic First Quarter, 2003.

Each student's set of scores for all the types of data provide a performance profile for the quarter. The student's individual profile may then be compared to the profiles of peers with the same or similar diagnoses and to the average score for all students in a particular school.

The AS students' name is stated for comparison purposes. The data indicate that the components of the program structure influence the performance of AS students positively, based on individual profiles of behavioral and academic performance. The data also indicate the AS student's gain when compared with non-AS peers.

This chapter has presented information about an approach to educating the student with AS. Examples of effective evidence-based instruction

Table 1. Measurement of Educational Goals (Cognitive)*

Goal	Evidenced by	Test item (illustrative)
1.0 Knowledge		
1.1 Knowledge of specifics	Recall of specific bits of information including terminology and specific facts such as definitions, events, dates, etc.	The Monroe Doctrine was announced about ten years after the: 1. Revolutionary War 2. War of 1812 3. Civil War 4. Spanish-American War
1.2 Knowledge of ways and means of dealing with specifics	Knowledge of ways of organizing, studying, and criticizing (conventions, trends and sequences, classifications, criteria, methodology)	Which of the following is a chemical change? 1. Evaporation of alcohol 2. Freezing of water 3. Burning of oil 4. Melting of wax 5. Mixing of sand and sugar
1.3 Knowledge of the universals and abstractions in a field	Knowledge of the major schemes and patterns by which phenomena and ideas are organized (principles and generalizations, theories and structures)	Some generalizations concerning the common metals are that: 1. most of the metals form only one insoluble salt 2. all the simple salts of the alkali metals are soluble 3. the metals of the alkaline earth group precipitated as carbonates 4. the alkali carbonates are insoluble in water 5. many of the heavy metal sulfides are insoluble in neutral or slightly acid solution
2.0 Comprehension		
2.1 Translation	Caro and accuracy with which a communication is paraphrased or rendered from one form (or language) of communication to another (understanding	"Milton! thou shouldst be leaving at this hour: England hath need of thee; she is a fen of stagnant waters" –Wordsworth. The metaphor, "she is a fen of

(continued)

* This table, showing the six cognitive levels identified by Benjamin S. Bloom, provides example of levels of academic tasks as each cognitive level. Although Bloom's taxonomy does not use the term "cognitive load," the table implies a higher load for tasks as higher cognitive levels and lower load at lower levels. Tasks above the level of "application" are problematic for students with AS.

Table 1. (*continued*)

Goal	Evidenced by	Test item (illustrative)
	of non-literal statements as well as translating verbal material into symbolic statements and vice versa).	stagnant waters," indicates that Wordworth felt that England was: 1. largely swampy land 2. in a state of turmoil and turmoil 3. making no progress in a generally corrupt condition
2.2 Interpretation	Explanation or summarization of a communication (grasping of the thought or major theme)	After presenting a paragraph or graph ask students to react to statements about the paragraph in the following manner: 1. if statement is *definitely* true 2. if statement is *probably* true 3. if the information given is not sufficient to indicate any degree of truth or falsity in the statement 4. if the statement is *probably* false 5. if the statement is *definitely* false
2.3 Extrapolation	Extension of trends or tendencies beyond the given data to determine implications, consequences, corollaries, effects, etc. (making of inferences and predictions)	Same as above
3.0 **Application**		
	Use of abstractions such as rules, principles, general ideas in particular, and concrete situation (solution of problems using concepts learned elsewhere).	The length of a rectangular lot exceeds its breadth by 20 yards. If each dimension is increased by 20 yards, the area of the lot will be doubled. Find the shorter dimension of the original lot. 1. 20 2. 30 3. 35 4. 40 5. none of the above
4.0 **Analysis**		
4.1 Analysis of elements	Identification of the elements involved in a communication.	A passage is presented in the test followed by the following

(*continued*)

Table 1. (*continued*)

Goal	Evidenced by	Test item (illustrative)
	(recognition of unstated assumptions, distinction between facts and hypotheses)	items: Which of the following is an *assumption*, specific to this experiment, that was made in the determination of the charge? 1. the force of gravity is the same whether the drops are charged or not 2. Opposite charges attract each other 3. Only a single charge is present on a drop 4. The mass of a drop is equal to its density times its volume

4.2 Analysis of members relationships	Identification of the connections and interactions between elements and parts of a communication (check of the consistency within a work and comprehension of interrelationships)	Family Income Percent of family
		Under $1,200 who received no medical
		1,200–3,000 *attention during the year*
		3,000–5,000 47
		5,000–10,000 40
		Over 10,000 33
		              24
		              14

		Conclusion: Members of families with small incomes are healthier than members of families with large incomes. Which of the following assumptions would be necessary to justify the conclusion? 1. Wealthy families had more money to spend for medical care 2. All members of families who needed medical attention received it 3. Many members of families with low incomes were not able to pay their doctor bills 4. Members of families with low incomes often did not receive medical attention
4.3 Analysis of organizational principles	Recognition of the organization, systematic arrangement, and structure which hold a	The theme of the musical selection presented is carried essentially by:

(*continued*)

Table 1. (*continued*)

Goal	Evidenced by	Test item (illustrative)
	communication together (recognition of form or pattern or techniques used)	1. the strings 2. the woodwinds 3. the horns 4. all in turn
5.0 Synthesis		
5.1 Production of a unique communication	Development of a novel communication which attempts to convey ideas, etc., to others (skill in writing or speaking)	Think of some time in your life when you were up against a difficulty, something that stood in your way and had to be overcome. Make up a story around this difficulty and tell it to the class.
5.2 Product of a plan or proposed set of operations	Development of a plan of work or the proposal of a plan of operations. (Proposal of ways to test hypothesis, production of a plan for accomplishing a goal)	Outline the steps that would be necessary to research the hypothesis that smoking is determinant of lung cancer.
5.3 Derivation of a set of abstract relations	Development of a set of abstract relations either to classify or explain particular data or phenomena, or the deduction of propositions and relations from a set of basic propositions or symbolic representations (formulation of appropriate hypotheses, making of generalizations)	After presenting data on a question, ask students to suggest relevant hypotheses and to indicate what additional data would be necessary to arrive at the "best" hypothesis.
6.0 Evaluation		
6.1 Judgments in terms of internal evidence	Determination of the accuracy, etc., of communication from such evidence as logical accuracy, consistency, documentation, etc.	Evaluate the following paragraph in terms of exactness of statement, documentation, proof, and logical consistency.
6.2 Judgments in terms of external criteria	Evaluation of material with reference to selected or remembered criteria. (comparison of major theories, facts, etc.; comparison of a work with the best known standards)	Write an essay evaluating the following poem. Your principles of evaluation should be made clear.

Source: Adapted from Benjamin S. Bloom (ed.) "Taxonomy of Educational Objectives" David McKay, Inc., New York, *Handbook I: Cognitive Domain*, 1956. For measurement of awareness, values, etc., see *Handbook II: Affective Domain*, 1964.

are discussed. We have noted the limits of current research and the lack of evidence for the efficacy of available information about teaching the AS student.

The chapter is organized to describe the AS student and his characteristics as they relate to classroom instruction. The typical classroom expectations of students are compared to the AS student's needs. Specific recommendations are made for optimal classroom modifications that will assist AS students to make social and academic performance gains.

Last, a model for assessing academic benefits provided one psychoeducational program is included with performance data of AS students and their non-AS peers.

The chapter is limited by the lack of information about prevocational and post-high school education, but such research remains unavailable. Longitudinal studies on the effect of early identification and intervention on the later development of AS students' academic and social skills remain sparse and anecdotal.

There is much work to be done in order to establish a hierarchy of developmental, social, and academic strategies that demonstrated success. Further research is needed on the student's ability to use skills learned in novel situations and the ability to generalize skills across settings.

Our preliminary research with pragmatic language assessment and remediation or habilitation indicates language patterns of AS students that are responsive to intervention. Further investigation is needed.

Last, TLC research on the relationship between levels of moral development in AS students and corresponding moral judgments and moral acts indicates a fertile set of issues for research.

The AS student who has a high level of intelligence and low level of social adaptability represents a significant challenge for education planners. These young people possess excellent intellectual potential and yet most fail to succeed in school and in independent living.

The AS student is a person for whom we must develop new knowledge and more effective advocacy.

References

Adreon, D., & Stella, J. (2001). Transition to middle and high school: increasing the success of students with asperger syndrome. *Intervention in School and Clinic, 36,* 266–271.

American Psychiatric Association. (1994). *Diagnostic and statistical manual of mental disorders* (4th ed.). Washington, DC: Author.

Barnhill, G., Hagiwara, T., Myles, B. S., & Simpson, R. L. (2000). Asperger syndrome: a study of the cognitive profiles of 37 children and adolescents. *Focus on Autism and Other Developmental Disabilities, 15,* 146–153.

Baron-Cohen, S., Wheelwright, S., Skinner, R., Martin, J., Clubley, E. (2001). The Autism-Spectrum Quotient (AQ): Evidene from Asperger Syndrome/High-Functioning Autism, Males and Females, Scientists and Mathematicians. *Journal of Autism and Developmental Disorders, 31*(1).

Bettison, S. (1996). The long-term effects of auditory training on children with autism. *Journal of Autism and Developmental Disorders, 26,* 361–374.

Burack, J. A. (1994). Selective attention deficits in persons with autism: Preliminary evidence of an attentional lens. *Journal of Abnormal Psychology, 103,* 3, 535–543.

Bloom, B. S. (ed.) (1956). *Taxonomy of Educational Objectives.* Handbook I: Cognitive Domain. New York: David McKay, Inc.

Bloom, B. S. (ed.) (1964). *Taxonomy of Educational Objectives.* (For measurement of awareness, values, etc.), Handbook II: Affective Domain. New York: David McKay, Inc.

Canivez, G. L., & Watkins, M. W. (1998). Long-Term Stability of the Wechsler Intelligence Scale for Children—Third Edition. *Psychological Assessment. 10,* 3, 285–291.

Church, C., Alisanski, S., & Amanulla, S. (2000). The social, behavioral, and academic experiences of children with asperger syndrome. Focus on Autism and Other Developmental Disabilities, *15,* 12–20.

Cognitive Load Theory (Winter 2003). *Educational Psychologist, 38.*

DuCharme, R. W., & McGrady, K. (2003a). *Pragmatic Skills Assessment & Social SkillsTraining for Students with Asperger Syndrome or High Functioning Autism.* MAAPS Conference, Westborough, MA.

DuCharme, R. W., & McGrady, K. (2003b). *Promoting the Healthy Development of Children with Asperger Syndrome: Education & Life Skills Issues.* Connecticut College, New London, CT.

DuCharme, R. W., & McGrady, K. (2002). *Social Skill Training and Pragmatic Skill Assessment forAsperger's Disorder or High Functioning Autism.* International Child & Adolescent Conference XI, Miami, FL.

DuCharme, R. W. (2001). *Asperger's Disorder: Differential Diagnosis Treatment Decisions and Treatment Effects Over Time.* MAAPS (Massachusetts Association of Approvied Private Schools) Conference, Marlborough, MA.

DuCharme, R. W. (1972). *Sight Word Acquisition Program.* Unpublished doctoral dissertation. University of Connecticut.

Fondacaro, D. (2001, February). Asperger syndrome:a qualitative study of successful educational interventions. Paper presented at the annual meeting of the Eastern Educational Research Association, Hilton Head, SC.

Frith, U. (1991). *Autism and Asperger syndrome.* New York: Cambridge University Press.

Ghaziuddin, M., & Gerstein, L. (1996). Pedantic speaking style differentiates asperger syndrome from high-functioning autism. *Journal of Autism and Developmental Disorders, 26,* 585–595.

Ghaziuddin, M., Weidmer-Mikhail, E., & Ghaziuddin, N. (1998). Comorbidity of Asperger syndrome: A preliminary report. *Journal of Intellectual Disability Research, 42*(4), 279–283.

Grace, D. (1998). *The Inclusion of Students with Emotional or Behavioral Disorders: What We Know About Effective and Non-Effective Practices.* Council for Children with Behavior Disorders, South East Regional Conference. May, Gulf Shores, AL.

Jackel, S. (1966). Asperger's Syndrome—Educational Management Issues.

Jolliffe, T., & Baron-Cohen, S. (1999). The strange stories test: A replication wit high-functioning adults with autism or asperger syndrome. *Journal of Autism and Developmental Disorders, 29,* 395–406.

Jones, R. S. P., & Meldal, T. O. (2001). Social Relationships and Asperger's syndrome. *Journal of Learning Disabilities, 5*(1), 35–41.

Kim, J. A., Szatmari, P., Bryson, S. E., Streiner, D. L., & Wilson, F. J. (2000). The prevalance of anxiety and mood problems among children with autism and asperger syndrome. *Autism: The International Journal of Research and Practice, 4,* 117–32.

Klin, A., Volkmar, F., & Sparrow, S. (2000). *Asperger Syndrome.* New York, NY: The Guilford Press.

Klin, A., Lang, J., Cicchetti, D. V., & Volkmar, F. R. (2000). *Brief Report: Interrater Reliability of Clinical Diagnosis and DSM-IV Criteria for Autistic Disorder: Results of the DSM-IV Autism Field Trial.*

Klin, A., Volkmar, F. R., Sparrow, S. S., Cicchetti, D. V. (1995). Validity and *neuropsychological characterization of Asperger Syndrome: Convergence with Nonverbal Learning Disabilities syndrome.* Journal of Child Psychology & Psychiatry & Applied Disciplines, *1127–1140.*

Koning, C., & Magill-Evans, J. (2001). Social and language skills in adolescent boys with asperger syndrome. *Autism: The International Journal of Research and Practice, 5,* 23–36.

Kunce, L., & Mesibov, G. B. (1998). Educational approaches to high-functioning autism and Asperger Syndrome. New York: Plenum.

Levine, M. (2002). *A Mind at a Time.* New York, NY: Simon & Schuster.

Little, L. (2001). Peer victimization of children with Asperger spectrum disorders. *Journal of the American Academy of Child & Adolescent Psychiatry, 40*(9), 995–996

Mayes, S. D., Calhoun, S. L., & Crites, D. L. (2001). Does DSM-IV Asperger Syndrome Exist? *Journal of Abnormal Child Psychology, 29*(3) 263–271.

Minshew, N. J., Meyer, J., Goldstein, G. (2002). Abstract reasoning in autism: A disassociation between concept formation and concept identification. *Neuropsychology.*

Neihart, M. (2000). Gifted children with asperger's syndrome. *Gifted Child Quarterly, 44,* 222–230.

Ozonoff, S., South, M., & Miller, J. (2000). DSM-IV defined Asperger syndrome: cognitive, behavioral and early history differentiation from high-functioning autism. *Autism: The International Journal of Research and Practice, 4,* 29–46.

Rinehart, N. J., Bradshaw, J. L., Brereton, A. V., & Tonge, B. J. (2002). Lateralization in individuals with high-functioning autism and Asperger's disorder. A frontostriatal model. *Journal of Autism & Developmental Disorders, 32*(4), 321–332.

Rinehart, N. J., Bradshaw, J. L., Moss, S. A., Brereton, A. V., & Tonge, B. J. (2001). A deficit in shifting attention present in high-functioning autism but no Asperger's disorder. *Autism,* Mar; 5(1): 67–80.

Rourke, B. P. (1995). *Syndrome of Nonverbal Learning Disabilities.* New York, NY: The Guilford Press.

Safran, S. P. (2001). Asperger Syndrome: The Emerging Challenge to Special Education. *The Council for Exceptional Children. 67*(2) 151–160.

Schopler, E., Mesibov, G. B., & Kunce, L. J. (1998). *Asperger Syndrome or High-functioning Autism?* New York, NY: Plenum Press.

Soderstrom, H., Rastrum, M., & Gillberg, C. (2002). Temperament and character in adults with asperger syndrome. *Autism: The International Journal of Research and Practice, 6,* 287–297.

Strain, P. S., & Schwartz, I. (2001). ABA and the development of meaningful social relations for young children with autism. *Focus on Autism and Other Developmental Disabilities, 16,* 120–128.

Sweller, J., & Chandler, P. (1991). Evidence for cognitive load theory. *Cognition and Instruction, 8,* 351–362.

Tantam, D. (2000). Psychological disorder in adolescents and adults with asperger syndrome. *Autism: The International Journal of Research and Practice, 4,* 47–62.

Tharpe, R. G., & Wetzel, R. J. (1969). *Behavior Modification in the Natural Environment*, New York: Academic Press, Inc.

Webster's New International Dictionary, Unabridged (1934). G. & C. Merriam Co.

Wing, L., & Gould, J. (1979). Severe impairments of social interaction and associated abnormalities in children, epidemiology and classification. *Journal of Autism and Developmental Disorders, 9*, 11–29.

Wing, L. (1988). The continuum of autistic characteristics. In E. Schopler & G.B. Mesibov (Eds.), *Diagnosis and assessment in autism* (pp. 91–111). New York: Plenum Press.

World Health Organization. (1992). *International Classification of diseases* (10th ed.). Geneva, Switzerland: Author.

Chapter 4

Counseling and Other Therapeutic Strategies for Children with Asperger Syndrome and Their Families

Ann Wagner and Kathleen A. McGrady

Introduction

Previous chapters have made it clear that the challenges of Asperger Syndrome (AS) lie in a developmental difference in the way individuals with the syndrome process information about social interactions and social relationships. Individuals with AS perceive and make sense of the world in ways that are unique, and these differences may be more or less subtle or obvious, depending on the situation. Additionally, there is evidence that cognitive differences are common if not universal. For example, there is a tendency to focus on details of information, often overlooking or failing to process the "big picture" and contributing to difficulty organizing complex information. People with AS are often tied to literal meanings of language so that they might have trouble with non-literal language such as metaphor or tone of voice. They often have a tendency to be inflexible,

The views expressed in this chapter are those of the authors and do not necessarily reflect the official position of the National Institute of Mental Health, the National Institutes of Health, or any other part of the U.S. Department of Health and Human Services. Mention of trade names, commercial products, or organizations does not imply endorsement by the U.S. Government.

both in terms of cognition and behavior, which can contribute to social and academic difficulty.

Previous chapters have described what we know about *how* this unique processing style occurs, and *what* can be done to help the individual overcome the difficulties he or she is likely to encounter. The chapters have, so far, stayed close to the common features of AS and the situations (e.g., social relationships and school performance) most uniformly and immediately affected by the unique way of perceiving and understanding the world that is typical of children with AS. In this chapter we want to expand the focus to include the family members and other caregiving relatives of an individual with AS. Additionally, there are times when the strain of managing the social and cognitive challenges result in secondary emotional problems such as anxiety and depression, which can impede adaptive functioning. This chapter will address what we know about treating these secondary symptoms when they arise.

As is true of all individuals, children with AS live, play, interact, and work in a world that is filled with people. While their "biology" might be the starting point for the challenges they face, the extent to which they can overcome these challenges depends to a large extent on the supports and resources that can be rallied to their assistance. For most children, and also for adults, the primary support network is the family. But, even when individuals with AS have the best support and care possible, the strain of their areas of disability can lead to adjustment problems or emotional distress. On the other hand, being a parent or caregiving relative of a child or adult with AS is in itself a challenge. There are several levels of support and assistance needed by families, from basic education about appropriate and effective interventions, to social and emotional support, to prevention of undue family stress or conflicts. Professional counseling can be integrated into an overall care plan for children with AS and their families to promote the best possible adjustment and prevent or ameliorate emotional distress.

It is important to consider the idea of "evidence-based" interventions. Within the field of health prevention and treatment, including mental health, there is a growing emphasis on promoting programs and treatments that have been scientifically "proven" to be effective (e.g., Lonigan et al., 1998; Rogers, 1998). Treatments that meet this level of proof are those that have been successfully compared with other treatments, using rigorous experimental methodology, and have been shown to be effective when replicated at sites other than the one where the treatment was developed. Rigorous methodology includes "controlled" conditions. That is, the study compares the effect of an intervention while controlling for other influences. Everything possible is done to be sure that there is not something else influencing the behavior in question. This might be done by controlling the timing of implementing and discontinuing a treatment (as in a single subject multiple baseline study), or by comparing two groups of individuals that differ only with regard to whether or not the treatment is applied (a controlled trial). Other techniques are needed to insure against bias by the experimenter or biased perceptions by the person evaluating the outcome. These include random assignment to a treatment group, having the investigators and subject "blind" to whether or not the individual is receiving the treatment, having evaluators of outcomes "blind" to the hypotheses of the study, and using standardized and reliable outcome measures rather than subjective reports of changes.

This scientific rigor is necessary for making reliable determinations of the efficacy of a treatment. It is, unfortunately, time-consuming and costly to conduct this type of research. When considering treatments for children with AS, there are very few interventions that would meet the criteria for being considered "evidence-based" by virtue of meeting this level of scientific scrutiny. That is not because nothing works, but it is because there have not been the kinds of rigorous studies needed for this level of scientific proof. This leaves professionals and parents with little evidence in either direction: that a treatment works, or that it doesn't work. This is the state of research on interventions in autism spectrum disorders in general. There is even less research that looks specifically at the how well treatment approaches work for children with AS.

In the sections below, we incorporate a review of the scientific evidence when it is available. Consistent with other chapters in this book, we will try to categorize interventions and treatment techniques according to "what works or probably works" meaning there is reasonable scientific evidence; "might work" based on theory and case report but has not been sufficiently tested; and "what doesn't work" meaning that the evidence is against it. Additionally, we draw on our own clinical backgrounds and experience with counseling children with AS and their families.

The reader has by now noticed some recurring themes in the discussions about helping children with AS:

- *Variability* in a particular child's development; with pronounced strengths and weaknesses
- *Variability* among children with AS; each child has a unique profile of strengths and challenges
- *Variability* in the child's adaptability and skills level, variability day-to-day and from one setting to another
- *Common challenges* faced by individuals with AS due to the underlying difficulties processing social information, predicting cause-and-effect relationships, and responding flexibly to the world around them

- The need for *structure and consistency* in the child's environment
- The assumption that failure to respond adaptively or appropriately to a situation usually reflects *skills deficits*, rather than intentional misbehavior, and calls for *skills-building* strategies
- One needs to differentiate between *skills deficits* and *performance deficits* before formulating an intervention strategy
- The need for *positive, nonjudgmental, nonpunitive* attitudes and strategies on the part of the adult helpers and caregivers

Another theme running throughout this book is the need to provide as much support and guidance as is necessary, while promoting self-regulation and self-sufficiency. In an ideal world, a child with AS would be assessed and evaluated early, intervention strategies would be tailored to his or her individual needs, the optimal level of assistance needed for skills development would be put into place, and there would be gradual movement from reliance on external support (the environment and care-givers) to self-sufficiency and self-reliance. This implies an individualized approach to intervention, as some children will need more imposed structure than others. One can imagine a continuum of intensity of externally-imposed structure, where self-contained special education classrooms and maximum levels of structure and routine at home represent one end of the continuum. At the other end might be full inclusion in a mainstream educational setting with minimal accommodations, and high levels of self-sufficiency at home. Many factors (e.g., age, cognitive and language ability, ability to self-monitor, internal emotional regulation, and availability of support resources) would contribute to the location along this continuum that would be optimal for a given individual.

Diagnosis as Intervention: Interpretation of the Child's Behavior within the Context of Asperger Syndrome

The Parent–Professional Diagnostic Team

Diagnosis and treatment of childhood disorders necessitates a team approach, where parents and professionals are partners in coming to the best possible understanding of the child and the best-informed decision about treatment strategies. Parents are absolutely crucial to this process. The developmental, medical, and family histories they provide are neces-sary components of a diagnosis. Their description of their child's behavior in a variety of settings is absolutely critical. The role of the professionals on the team is to interpret the information parents can provide within the context of what is known about AS. Details about the components of an appropriate evaluation and diagnosis can be found in several sources, such as *The World of the Autistic Child* by Bryna Siegel (1996); the chapter by Ami Klin and colleagues on "Assessment Issues in Children and Adolescents with AS" in *Asperger Syndrome* (Klin et al., 2000); "Practice Parameters for the Assessment and Treatment of Children, Adolescents, and Adults with Autism and Other Pervasive Disorders" (American Academy of Child and Adolescent Psychiatry, 1999).

The first task of the parent-professional team is to come to a mutual understanding of the experiences and behavior of a child with AS. To come to the best understanding possible, the experience and knowledge the parent has of his or her child should be combined with an expert's knowledge about the characteristics common to individuals with AS. The importance of this mutual understanding cannot be overstated. Parents often arrive at the AS diagnosis after several attempts to understand the difficulties their child is having. Because children with AS often have a puzzling combination of strengths and difficulties, and because they often have behaviors or symptoms similar to those found in other disorders (e.g., attention problems, anxiety, learning disabilities), identification and diagnosis is often not straightforward. Sometimes parents ask for evaluations because they know something is amiss, but because on the surface cognitive and language skills appear to be intact, they are told that nothing is wrong. It is also common for a child to accumulate a series of symptom-specific diagnoses (e.g., ADHD, anxiety disorder, oppositional disorder) without any explanation of the "bigger picture" or why all of these symptoms are clustering within one child. And occasionally there are blatant mis-diagnoses when the social deficits are misunderstood and the child's unusual behaviors or utterances (e.g., self-talk, reference to fantasy or cartoon figures, or imaginary friends) are interpreted as signs of psychosis or antisocial behavior; or assumptions are made about abuse or other environmental causes for the behavior. The time that elapses between initial concern and obtaining diagnosis and treatment is often several years. This protracted delay must be avoided, and we must be better at making the diagnosis and providing appropriate, individualized treatment.

That said, this mutual understanding might not occur immediately. For many reasons, the professionals' conceptualization of the situation may not be compatible with the parents' view. In this case, an extended dialogue may be necessary, and follow-up visits to discuss further the diagnosis and recommendations may be needed. The professional team should be honest and straightforward about their opinion, while respectful of that of the parents. Often, if all parties are respectful and open-minded, minor disagreements about labels can be tabled while appropriate interventions are pursued. Parents might want to pursue a "second opinion" and should feel free to do so. Except for the very rare instance in which a child is being harmed, or a delay in attaining intervention puts the child's safety at risk, it is best to take the time necessary to keep open an ongoing dialogue and come to a mutual understanding.

In our experience, despite the fact that having a diagnosis of AS is not "good" news, parents are quite relieved if they come to a better understanding of their child's condition. That in itself is good intervention, because it allows parents to shed feelings of responsibility and inadequacy, helps them understand that challenging behavior is usually not intentional, and helps them respond in a more facilitative way when their child is having trouble.

The diagnostic team is usually composed of several professionals, although the exact team can vary. Commonly, a child psychologist (e.g., clinical psychologist, developmental psychologist or neuropsychologist), speech/language pathologist and possibly a physician (child psychiatrist, pediatrician, or neurologist) compose the core of professionals. Depending on the setting, educators, occupational therapists, social workers, physical therapists, or others may also be involved in the process. The process of delivering the results of all of these pieces of the assessment deserves careful thought and planning. Difficulties at home, school, and other settings need to be addressed. Sometimes, parents meet individually with each professional, get results piecemeal and are left on their own to integrate the various findings. At the other extreme is the meeting in which parents sit with a room full of professionals and are given detail after detail of the types of tests administered and results. Parents are then allowed to ask questions. But, one can easily see that after being bombarded with this much information, with little time to digest it, even formulating a question would be a challenge.

We propose two alternative scenarios, which although untested and unproven, have worked well in our experience. In an *integrated interpretive session*, after a case conference with all professional team members present, two or three key members of the evaluation team meet with the parents or primary caregivers to discuss results of the evaluation. An hour and a half is a reasonable amount of time to allow for full discussion of the evaluation results and time for parents to ask questions. In this model, the information is discussed and integrated with the parents so all team members come away with the same picture. Deciding on intervention strategies is a cooperative effort between the parents and key professionals. This scenario is obviously time-intensive and costly in terms of professional time. Although we believe that parents deserve this level of effort, it is not always possible. Alternatively, a *case conference/case management* model can be applied. In this scenario, the evaluation team holds a case conference with all team members present to discuss, integrate, and interpret the evaluation results. The team also determines intervention recommendations. A designated member of the team becomes the case manager, and meets with the parents to discuss the evaluation results and recommendations.

Parents know the individual child better than anyone, but professionals have a "broad view" of what is normative or typical and where this child might differ from that. Mutual respect for the expertise of the other will result in the best treatment. Nevertheless, professionals have to keep in mind that the parents have the ultimate responsibility for their children. Before agreeing to a treatment or intervention approach, parents should be comfortable with it, and should feel that the approach makes sense for their particular child. There is a lot of ambiguity in the process of diagnosing AS and developing an intervention program. As children grow, the situations and challenges they face change, and so their supports must anticipate and respond to these changing needs. At any given time in a child's life, there may be several members of his or her "treatment team": a counselor, a teacher, a tutor, a speech/language therapist, a pediatrician, or others.

Ongoing Consultation for Monitoring and Decision-Making

Parents often like to have an ongoing relationship with a trusted professional consultant who can help them navigate through the changes that occur as their child grows and develops. A professional with expertise in AS, who also becomes very familiar with a particular child and family, can be helpful as decisions have to be made about schools, or medications, or helping the child adjust to new social situations. Where does a family find such a consultant? Often during the lengthy course of obtaining a diagnosis and intervention plan, the parents develop a particularly trusting relationship with one team member who is able to serve in this capacity. Alternatively, as they get to know their community they may identify such a person, perhaps recommended by another parent or member of the treatment team, who can be sought out particularly for this role as consultant. The consultant's profession or degree is not crucial. The development of AS as a professional specialty happens in the context of many disciplines. Psychologists, pediatricians, educators, psychiatrists, speech/language pathologists, social workers, and nurses can and have become experts in the field. Similarly, no particular degree or profession guarantees that the individual has experience or expertise in this area. At this time, the development of expertise in autism spectrum disorders, including AS, is something that an individual pursues beyond the training needed to obtain their professional credentials. The level of experience and expertise, and the rapport with the child's family, are the critical elements in this partnership.

Comprehensive Treatment Programs: The Right Choice for Asperger Syndrome?

One of the first decisions parents must make after their child receives a diagnosis of AS is how and when to intervene. Armed with the results of a comprehensive assessment and recommendations from a treatment team, they must determine what resources are available and appropriate for their child. It is always wise to find out what can be provided by the public school system. The Individual with Disabilities Education Act (IDEA) assures a "free and appropriate" public education to "children" ages 3–21 who have been diagnosed with learning disabilities. IDEA specifically covers autistic disorder, but whether or not AS is covered depends on the particular state's definition of disabilities. The quality and extent of services that are provided are variable from one community to another, even within a particular school district. Parents will want to ask advice of trusted professionals or parents of other children with similar difficulties who are familiar with local services.

Numerous comprehensive early intervention programs for children with autism and PDD have been developed and described (National Research Council, 2001; Rogers, 1998; Dawson & Osterling, 1997; Hurth et al., 1999). Programs described in these publications are listed in the appendix at the end of the chapter. The National Research Council (2001) provides descriptions of 10 model programs that were considered representative of well-described, and well-respected comprehensive treatment programs. None of these programs has been rigorously tested to the extent that one could say with confidence that "it works". The program that comes closest to attaining this level of evidence is the UCLA Young Autism Project (Lovaas, 1987; McEachin et al., 1993; Sheinkopf & Siegel, 1998; Smith et al., 2000), although there remain questions about for whom it works best, and the intensity necessary for treatment success.

None of these programs has been evaluated specifically for effectiveness with children with AS. Although there is no reason to believe that the techniques would be less effective, there is some evidence that the same level of intensity may not be necessary for "higher functioning" children with autism spectrum disorders, or children without mental retardation, and this would include children with AS (Sheinkopf & Siegel, 1998; Smith, 1999). Intensive, comprehensive early intervention programs may or may not be appropriate for a child with AS. As a group, children with AS have better cognitive and language abilities than do most children with Autism, for whom these programs were developed. They often are better able to participate in less intensive intervention programs, or mainstream educational programs with varying degrees of support. By definition, children with AS do not have mental retardation. They may be within the "typical" range of intelligence or have IQ well above average. Intervention decisions depend on the child's unique developmental profile, as well as the family's values and resources.

Some questions parents might want to ask when considering treatment programs, whether private or publicly funded, are listed below.

- How successful has the program been for children like mine, with the same diagnosis, similar age, and similar developmental profile?
- Has the program itself been evaluated for effectiveness with children with AS? If not, are the techniques used based on models and/or theory that have some scientific validation?
- How does the program attempt to move children toward more self-sufficiency and less restrictive educational settings?
- Are staff members trained to work with children with AS? What is the extent of their training?
- How will my child's goals and progress be measured?
- What are the cost, time commitment, and location of the program?

Psychoeducation and Consultation with Families and Other Primary Caregivers

There are several models of family support and intervention. None have been "tested" specifically with families of individuals with AS. Some have been evaluated for families with children with autism. Because families' needs vary, the decision about what type of support is needed, and when, is made based on family preference and family need.

Psychoeducation

Psychoeducation refers to the provision of information related to psychological conditions. Components often include condition-specific information, information on community support services, legal information (e.g., rights, entitlements, and relevant public laws), and a discussion of life transitions and future needs. There may also be skills training to help parents interact more effectively with family members, teachers, and professionals. This information can be delivered to an individual, family, or in a group format.

Psychoeducational models have been shown to be helpful as a component of comprehensive mental health intervention packages for chronic mental health conditions such as bipolar disorder and schizophrenia (Penn & Mueser, 1996; Miklowitz et al., 2000). Although not evaluated for usefulness with families of children with AS, there are parallels (e.g., lifelong challenges, effect on family members, need for multiple sources of support) that suggest a similar model may be beneficial. While the need for providing information to families about diagnosis, prognosis and resources seems obvious, the timing and mode of delivery are important. Information should always be provided to parents at the time of diagnosis, of course, and coming to an understanding of the disorder and its causes can be helpful for managing the emotional impact of learning that one's child probably faces a lifetime of challenges. On the other hand many, if not most, families report mental and emotional "overload" around the time of their child's evaluation and diagnosis, making it hard to retain information or think of all of the questions they would like to ask. Psychoeducation should not be considered a "one-shot" activity. There need to be several sources of opportunity for obtaining information, including follow-up appointments in the diagnostic clinic, occasional informational group meetings, and special meetings with families around times of transition and decision-making. Giving parents written material is especially helpful, as it allows them to read or re-read information as questions arise, or as new challenges emerge. The responsibility for providing timely, appropriate information is a shared one: shared by the diagnostic clinic, school, and other major service providers.

Parent Support Groups

Parent support groups are almost as varied as the families that participate in them. They almost always involve some degree of psychoeducation, as well as a source for information about local resources. They vary with regard to the expectation for intimate sharing of emotions and personal information. Some groups are organized and moderated by parents, others are led by professionals. There are no guidelines for determining what type of group is best for what type of parent. In fact, some parents do not find groups helpful at all, and might opt out. So, while support groups can be extremely helpful sources of information and support, parents should not feel obligated to join one. There need to be alternative ways for obtaining the information and resources available.

Web-based resources and chat rooms are an alternative to support groups. This might be the best option for parents who are uncomfortable with groups or who cannot attend group meetings for logistical reasons. Several sources of good information are available on line.

Support groups and online resources are efficient ways to impart important information and resources. Most are very careful about the types of information they are disseminating and thoughtful about the impact the content and interactions might have on group members or website visitors. However, there is no oversight of support groups and there seldom is scientific screening of the information being presented in a group or over the internet. Parents should approach these resources as "informed consumers". They should find out the credentials of the group leaders or owners of the web sites. They should ask questions about the resources and recommendations being promoted. If in doubt, consultation with a professional should always be undertaken.

Facilitating Parent-Child Interactions: Methods Specific to Autism Spectrum Disorders

BEHAVIORAL PARENT TRAINING.   Methods based on "applied behavior analysis" or ABA for teaching skills and facilitating more appropriate and adaptive behaviors are widely used. ABA methods have also been extensively tested for their effectiveness with children with autism and other developmental disabilities (e.g., Lovaas, 1987; McEachin et al., 1993; Sheinkopf & Siegel, 1998; Smith et al., 2000, Dunlap & Fox, 2001). This mode of intervention is the only one that could be said to have accumulated enough scientific evidence that most would agree that "it works" in children with autism spectrum disorders. ABA, and comprehensive programs based on applied behavioral analysis, are based on the principle that when a behavior is rewarded it is likely to be repeated. Behaviors that are not rewarded, or that result in an undesirable consequence, tend to gradually go away. By carefully analyzing the causes and consequences of a particular behavior, identifying an opposite, competing behavior (desired behavior) and consistently altering the consequences so that they reward the desired behavior, one can teach new skills or transform inappropriate behaviors into more acceptable ones. This relatively simple principle has been developed into techniques that have been shown to be highly effective for teaching new skills, increasing the frequency of appropriate or adaptive behaviors, and decreasing the frequency of inappropriate or maladaptive behaviors.

How and when to apply these techniques, however, requires careful consideration. It is very important that behaviors are taught that have the potential to generalize to other settings. For instance, teaching a child to make eye contact with a speech therapist is of limited use unless the child also makes eye contact when conversing with parents, peers, and others. One way to increase generalization is to help parents reinforce and apply the behavioral techniques at home and in the community. For this reason, good behavioral programs always contain a parent-training component.

Additionally, when parents are taught how to apply behavioral techniques, with ongoing coaching, they can be effective in smoothing out interactions between the child with AS and his or her family members. These techniques work best when applied to very specific behaviors to teach (e.g., waiting one's turn in a conversation) or change (e.g., being more cooperative at bedtime). When parents feel effective, when there is less conflict between the parent and child, and when the child is able to function more adaptively in the community, the relationship between parent and child improves. Behavioral techniques can also be used to work on very specific social behaviors, such as making appropriate greetings, appropriate modes of expressing affection, sharing, and playing interactively.

Parents are most likely to learn applied behavior analysis techniques when enrolling their children in a comprehensive treatment program. As these comprehensive treatment programs have evolved, there has been a trend toward teaching parents to implement the programs, and toward utilizing the behavior management techniques in more naturalistic settings and during typical activities, and toward developing goals based on the child's unique developmental profile (Ingersoll et al., 2001). There is also a trend, at least when applied to programs for children and adults with developmental disabilities, away from emphasizing the consequences of a behavior to an emphasis on understanding the triggers of a behavior, proactively providing cues or rehearsal of the appropriate behavior, making changes in the environment to avoid or minimize those triggers, and teaching more adaptive or appropriate responses when the triggers cannot be avoided (for example, "stop and separate" strategies such as time-outs). A large body of literature, based mostly on the accumulation of single-subject and small-case design studies, provides cumulative support for these techniques. A comprehensive review of this literature, and practical guidance for implementation can be found in *Positive Behavioral Support: Including People with Difficult Behavior in the Community* (Koegel et al., 1996).

There are also comprehensive treatment programs that derive strategies from a developmental theoretical framework. For instance, the Denver Model (Rogers et al., 2000) emphasizes the need to establish interpersonal relationships as a foundation to achieving other developmental milestones, and so emphasizes the social and emotional aspects of social relatedness. The Developmental Intervention Model (Greenspan & Wieder, 1997) is based on an assumption that the social problems in autism spectrum disorders is caused by abnormal or atypical processing of sensory information and difficulties with emotional regulation. The focus is on addressing sensory processing irregularities and the establishment of emotional contact. Both of these programs place heavy emphasis on improving parent-child relationships. While most of these programs have not been extensively evaluated using rigorous scientific trials, there are theoretical reasons and some preliminary scientific evidence that they can be useful for many children with autism spectrum disorders (Rogers, 1998; National Research Council, 2001), and presumably for some children with AS. Many well-established programs combine elements of behavioral and developmental orientations (TEACCH: Marcus et al., 2000; Walden Program: McGee et al., 2000). Some have specifically evaluated the effectiveness of the parent training components of their programs. Parent training models that are promising based on evidence provided by their developers include the LEAP Program (Strain & Cordisco, 1994), the Denver Model (Rogers et al., 2000), the Individualized Support Program at the University of South Florida (Dunlap, 1999) and the Pivotal Response Training Model (Koegel et al., 1999), and the Douglas Developmental Center Program (Harris et al., 2000). Whatever the theoretical underpinning, well-established and effective programs always include an emphasis on the parent-child relationships and overall family support (Dawson & Osterling, 1997). Furthermore, there is evidence that parents can learn to employ these methods and that doing so helps them feel better in general, and more satisfied and confident in their parenting role (Koegel et al., 1996; Ozonoff & Cathcart, 1998, Schreibman 1997, Sofronoff & Farbotko, 2002).

If a child is not involved in a comprehensive treatment program such as the one described above, parents may not have automatic access to professionals who can teach them behavioral techniques. Parents should be informed of options for accessing this type of assistance. Local chapters of support networks, schools, intervention specialists, and diagnostic specialists should be knowledgeable about local resources. Of particular need is access to support for behavioral issues across the lifespan, especially during transition out of the care of the education system and into independent living.

A cautionary note is in order for parents who are looking for behavior management training. Several good parent training programs have been developed and packaged for managing difficult child behaviors, and are often implemented in community settings. They generally focus on increasing the child's cooperation with parents' requests and improving family relationships. They do not necessarily focus on the types of social misunderstanding, communication problems, and inflexibility that are inherent in children with AS. Parents should be careful, then, to find out whether these aspects will be addressed in the program, and whether the trainer has expertise with Asperger syndrome.

Family Therapy

There is no reason to believe that as a group the families of children with AS are any different from most families. Having a family member with a developmental or learning disorder is, however, a stressor for all families. Lee Marcus and colleagues (1997) at the TEACCH Program list unique stressors experienced by families of children with autism spectrum disorders, most of which apply to AS in general. These include being exposed to lengthy confusion or disagreement about the diagnosis; the uneven and unusual course of development; trying to determine what behaviors are related to inability versus unwillingness; public behavior which is sometimes embarrassing to parents and siblings; differences of opinion among professionals; and the constant surfacing of fads and unproven therapies. Additionally, the process of educating and teaching parents behavior management techniques can have an impact on the family system (Harris & Powers, 1984).

Raising a child who may need supervision and guidance throughout the lifespan raises critical issues for decision-making and family planning. Protection against consequences of social misunderstanding (e.g., victimization) have to be thought through with an eye toward immediate as well as long term safety. Parents will have to decide whether or not to place limits on independent decision-making when it comes to issues such as driving, managing money, sexual behavior/birth control, and living alone. Issues of trusts and guardianship or conservatorship have to be considered.

Most families adjust well. They may have to reformulate their priorities or make adjustments to their lifestyles. They often are able to identify positive outcomes, such as a renewed appreciation for family. Nevertheless, stress can exacerbate vulnerabilities in a family system, and this can show up as strain in other family relationships, such as strain between parents, conflict between siblings, or parent-child conflicts (with the unaffected child). Taking a systems view is necessary (Harris & Powers, 1984), and professionals should be prepared to institute family therapy or refer the family to an experienced family therapist, if it is needed.

Counseling and Therapeutic Strategies for the Child or Adolescent with Asperger Syndrome

Some individuals with AS adapt remarkably well with little specialized professional help. Innate ability and the availability of intuitive, nurturing adults undoubtedly helps (see chapter by S. Shore in this book for an example). Most, however, are in need of some level of guidance throughout the school years and into adulthood. Even those who can survive without knowledgeable, professional assistance, might find life easier with the support of someone who recognizes the syndrome and the challenges inherent in it.

As children move along the continuum toward increasing self-reliance, there is a need for ongoing coaching and assistance with problem-solving. If the child is in school, it is particularly useful if this person is within the school system. A school counselor, social worker, speech therapist, or others, can provide regularly scheduled counseling sessions, intervene early to prevent a problem from becoming a crisis, and facilitate communication among the teachers and other school personnel. At times, it may be appropriate for a professional outside of the school system to provide ongoing counseling or therapy. The caveat here, though, is that this person will have to remain in close communication with parents, teachers, and other individuals who are also providing guidance to the child. The need for continuity cannot be stressed enough, and the child will need the support of adults in his or her "natural" environment in order to generalize skills learned in a professional's office to the real world. The following sections describe strategies for providing support to the child with Asperger Disorder.

Interactional Style: A Key Ingredient for Maintaining a Positive Relationship

If one considers carefully the ways in which children with AS process information, especially social information, one arrives at a blueprint for interaction that avoids or at least minimizes the "land mines" of social interaction that are common. For example, we know that people with AS have difficulty attending to the salient aspects of a social situation, that they have difficulty understanding nuances and integrating multiple sources of information. They may be under-reactive or over-reactive to the affect of others, but in either case they are likely to have difficulty understanding the cause of the emotion. They are likely to misjudge the impact their behavior has on others. They are easily overwhelmed by complex information and may need extra time to process and respond. It is, therefore, helpful to keep interactions and communications simple and straightforward, try to maintain neutral affect, explain one's actions and check for understanding, and allow extra time for processing and responding.

Below are guidelines used at The Learning Clinic. These guidelines are written for school personnel, but can easily be adapted for professionals outside of the school, as well as for parents.

INTERACTIONAL STYLES FOR WORKING WITH
ASPERGER/PDD STUDENTS

Visual Strategies

Cue cards
Color Cues
Templates

Multi-Sensory Learning

It is always helpful to incorporate as many sensory modalities as possible – visual, auditory, tactile (touch), taste, and smell. For example, use the sense of touch by having students handle task-related objects, and also include movement when appropriate. Pair verbal instruction with visual charts, lists, or pictures.

Executive Functioning Help

Cognitive organization: Functional Writing Model
Task levels: Bloom's Cognitive Levels (Knowledge, Comprehension, Application)

Off-Task

Self-selected task options are typically reinforcing (use agreed upon standards prior to starting tasks).
Establish clear task expectations, performance requirements, rehearsal strategies, and checks.
Provide short breaks between tasks
Nonverbal cue: tap on the shoulder
Verbal cue: quietly call student's name and redirect to task

Self-Stimulation Behaviors

Verbal cue: Call student by name, and then clearly direct student back to his task. Use competing behavior model as part of redirection

(continued)

Voice of Staff

1. Student responds more positively when spoken to in a mild/moderate tone of voice. It is important to practice consistently using this tone of voice.
2. Avoid any use of sarcasm, vague, or undirected general comments.

Proximity

1. Maintain appropriate proximity, and do not give verbal direction outside of a 3' to 4' distance from student.
2. Require acknowledgment of the direction given.

Directions

1. Student requires additional time to process information before making a response. Therefore, when giving student a direction or transitioning student from one activity to another, include the following modifications:
   a. Provide concrete directions.
   b. Always provide *extra time for processing* the information/request, before the student is expected to comply with the direction.
   c. *Verify the student's understanding* of the direction by asking student to repeat his understanding of the directions in his own words.
   d. Break down request into no more than two steps at a time.
   e. When appropriate to the situation, provide written step-by-step directions (in additional to the verbal) to which the student can refer.

Activities and Transitions

1. Advance, multiple rehearsals of activities and transitions are essential for success. This includes Daily Plans, class group activities, and any transitions/changes to routine.
   a. Provide concrete information.
   b. Always provide *extra processing time* (10–20 seconds).
   c. At each rehearsal, *verify the student's understanding* of the information by asking student to repeat his understanding of the information in his own words.
   d. Break down information into no more than two steps at a time.
   e. When appropriate to the situation, provide written step-by-step directions (in additional to the verbal) to which the student can refer.
   f. Provide multiple advance (weeks, days, hours) rehearsals of impending activities/transitions.

(continued)

g. Again, on the day of the activity/transition, rehearse student on what will happen.

h. Prior to the activity/transition, again rehearse the student, and *provide extra processing time* before he is expected to start the activity/process of transitioning—ending the current task, and beginning the next.

i. Provide time for review of past information, review tests, verbal restatements.

Time-Off Space

Always identify in advance the area where student can take a time-off. This will be the student's "safe space." When he becomes agitated/frustrated, student should take a time-off in the agreed upon area. If he does not initiate it, direct him to take a time-out.

It is important that the time-off be taken in a different area—change of environment/stimulus that is contributing to the agitation. It is *not* effective to simply stop a task and take a time-off in the same area.

Sensory Overload

Signs of Sensory Overload

1. Anxious behaviors
2. Perseverates—gets "stuck" on a topic, or behavior
3. Nonsequitors—making statements that are unrelated to the task or current conversation
4. Off-task—inability to sustain attention and concentration
5. Rude
6. Aggressive behavior

Preventative Strategies

1. To prevent emotional and behavioral decompensation secondary to sensory overload, it is essential to first identify the antecedents.
   a. identify antecedents
   b. problem-solve how to minimize/eliminate the sensory overload.

(continued)

Functional Analysis: A Basis for Intervention Planning

Difficulty understanding and responding to social information is the unifying characteristic of people with AS. However, the severity of this difficulty and the manner in which it is expressed is variable. Furthermore,

c. provide rehearsal of expected (appropriate) behavior.

d. Provide *extra processing time* (10–20 seconds).

2. Voice modulation (staff)

Always speak to student in a calm manner.

Never use loud volume, or angry tone.

3. When teaching novel concepts, use:

a. hands on practice (concrete experiences)

b. incorporate multiple sensory modalities (*pair verbal with visual, tactile, kinesthetic, taste, smell*). Also use colors and sound.

4. Provide context ("Big Picture"). For example:

a. present information in a story context

b. create associations between bits of information

c. help draw conclusions (cause and effect—if this, then that)

d. differentiate the relevant from irrelevant

Reactive Strategies

If student is frustrated or agitated (early signs of emotional/behavioral decompensation), provide a Sensory Integration Break.

1. Direct student to separate from the situation, (e.g. time-out, outdoor physical activity)

a. direct student to his "safe space."

b. or, student may be directed to an outdoor physical activity (e.g. walking, playing basketball, etc.)

3. After student is emotionally and behaviorally stable, provide external support.

a. Help student process what happened

i. Identify the trigger. Determine what is overloading him.

ii. Provide clarification, support, etc.

iii. problem-solve how to minimize/eliminate the sensory overload

iv. help the student interpret the interaction

1. identify the appropriate social/behavioral response for which the situation called

2. staff can role-model the expected behavior

the child's emotional ability is only one component of a highly individual pattern of strengths and weaknesses. If a child is able to manage his or her challenges without difficulty, either in the form of internal distress or conflict with others, there is no need to intervene. Usually, however, the child with AS does encounter situations that either cause unhappiness and stress, or cause others to be unhappy with his or her behavior. Then, one has to determine what is the underlying cause of this particular child's difficulty.

An important first step for addressing social and behavioral difficulties is an accurate assessment to identify areas of weakness, as well as areas of strength. Knowing what a student cannot do is essential to determine *what* skill is lacking. However, identifying areas of strength provides information about *how* we can go about building the skill or developing compensatory strategies. Appendix A is an example of a Functional Analysis method (Maag & Reid, 1994) that has been adapted for use with youngsters with AS at The Learning Clinic. It is used to ascertain skill level in the social, cognitive, and behavioral domains and provides a comprehensive assessment of skills in each of these areas. Again, while was designed for use by school personnel, it could easily be adapted by other consultants and taught to parents for use in the home.

Social Skills and Communication Training

Social skills and communication skills are inextricably interwoven. The child with AS has difficulty in both areas, and interventions must include both. The examples of social skills instruction provided in the chapter by Dr. Brenda Smith Myles demonstrate this concept. Although additional information about social skills instruction is not needed here, it is worth emphasizing the important role of communication, and the particular vulnerabilities that children and youth with AS possess in this area.

Although "typically developing language" is a prerequisite for a diagnosis of AS, there are often specific weaknesses in language processing and language use even though the child started using words and sentences at an appropriate age. While the child with AS may have an exceptional vocabulary, and basically intact structural language skills, they often have difficulty with comprehension. Their understanding of the nuances of the words they use may be more impaired than is immediately apparent. Organizational deficits contribute both to misunderstanding of complex verbal input, as well as difficulty expressing oneself coherently. Pragmatic language (the social use of language) is universally impaired in individuals with AS, and they often do not appreciate that communication patterns are different with different people (such as the difference in style when talking with peers versus with adults). Yet again, because of the vast variability in skills among these individuals, the exact nature of a particular child's pragmatic skills needs to be evaluated, and the results need to be taken into account when planning instruction and intervention techniques. Appendix B is a description of The Learning Clinic's Pragmatic Skills Survey (DuCharme, 1992).

At TLC, the analysis of pragmatic skills strengths and weaknesses is incorporated into an intervention plan, and an Adult Mentor is used to facilitate these skills with peers. An example of a treatment plan for integrating pragmatic language and social skills building is below.

SKILL BUILDING STRATEGIES

1. Provide Adult Mentor to:
   a. *interpret* social situations—What behavior is being asked for? What is the appropriate verbal or behavioral response to this particular situation?
   b. *role model* the appropriate verbal or behavioral response
2. Role model perspective-taking
   Interpret for student the other person's intent, feelings, etc.
3. Role model the following:
   a. *entry* and *exit* statements of social communication
   b. competitive vs. aggressive behaviors
   c. assertive vs. rude statements/behaviors
   d. assertive vs. threatening statements/behaviors
4. 4. Provide opportunity for student to practice the following. Initially with Adult Mentor; then with peers (one at a time, then small groups):
   a. *entry* and *exit* statements of social communication
   b. voice modulation
   c. competitive vs. aggressive behaviors
   d. assertive/polite vs. rude statements/behaviors
   e. assertive vs. threatening statements/behaviors
5. Videotape role-playing scenarios for all of the above, and provide video feedback.
6. Provide opportunity for practice in "real life" settings, and provide feedback

---

There is a fairly large literature on social skills intervention for children with autism (see Rogers 2000 for a thorough review), but it is not clear which of the techniques are appropriate and effective for children with AS. If one extrapolates from the literature on social skills instruction with high-functioning children with autism, there are some techniques that seem to have potential. Use of videotape modeling to teach conversation skills has been used successfully, provided that the modeling is followed by live practice sessions with an adult (Charlop & Milstein, 1989). Peer-tutoring techniques (Kamps et al., 1994; Dugan et al., 1995) have been shown to increase social engagement as well as improve academic skills. Group-based social skills instruction has had mixed outcomes, with some evidence of improved social skills and generalization across settings in school-age children with high-functioning autism (Kamps et al., 1992), but others have not been able to demonstrate generalization in adolescents after group social skills instruction (Ozonoff & Miller, 1995). Some creative and interesting techniques based on pivotal response therapy have been reported, including the use of high-functioning children's preoccupations as a basis for invented games to engage peers in play (Baker et al., 1998) and teaching self-management strategies for social behaviors such as appropriate eye contact and maintaining a conversational topic (Koegel & Frea, 1993).

Authors with extensive clinical experience with youth with AS (e.g., DuCharme, in press; Myles in press; Mesibov et al., 2001; Klin & Volkmar, 2000) agree with the major components of social skills instruction:

- Problem-solving skills and strategies must be explicitly taught
- Generalization techniques must be built in
- Social awareness and social skills training should be integrated into all aspects of the child's education and therapy
- Reading social cues is essential to being able to respond flexibly and appropriately
- Social use of language (pragmatic skill) is central to successful social interaction
- Self-evaluation and self-monitoring should be fostered; a realistic assessment of one's own strengths and weaknesses is important
- Use of visual strategies to support concepts can be helpful, although care must be taken when using them with children with visual-spatial weaknesses.

Finally, Rogers (2000) makes an important distinction between social behavior and quality of social relationships. We don't know whether teaching more appropriate social interaction skills is sufficient for fostering more satisfying friendships and/or family relationships. As the literature on teaching social and communication skills develops, there is a need for determining how these techniques impact overall quality of relationships, and for determining what other variables might be important.

Counseling and Other Forms of Individual Psychotherapy for Youth with Asperger Syndrome

Although individual counseling or therapy is not likely to sufficiently address the core social difficulties of an individual with AS, there are situations in which it can be helpful. Given the challenges they face every day, and the potential for inadvertently ending up in conflict with others around them, the potential for developing stress-related symptoms of anxiety, sadness, loneliness, or maladaptive preoccupations is high. Although there are no population-based estimates of comorbid psychological disorders in individuals with AS, some research suggests a higher-than-typical rate of depression and anxiety in children and adolescents with AS (Muris, et al., 1998; Gillott et al., 2001; Klin et al., 1995; Kim et al., 2000). Certainly, case reports, professional books and manuals, and first-hand accounts provide evidence that anxiety, preoccupations, and depression are very common.

Cognitive behavior therapy (CBT) has strong evidence of efficacy in treating anxiety, depression, and obsessive/compulsive symptoms in children without developmental disorders (see Hibbs & Jensen, 1996, for reviews of CBT applications). CBT addresses distorted cognitions, teaches self-awareness and emotional awareness, and problem solving. These cognitive techniques seem to be consistent with the types of strategies proposed for teaching other kinds of adaptive skills to children with autism spectrum disorders. There is one case report of successful treatment of an adult with high-functioning autism and depression, using a modified version of CBT. Many versions of manualized CBT are available, and further investigation of this model for treating individuals with AS would be beneficial to the field.

Medication for Secondary Symptoms Commonly Associated with Asperger Syndrome

Medication is often used to treat behavior problems and emotional symptoms in children and youth with autism spectrum disorders. Martin et al. (2000) surveyed 109 children, adolescents and adults with high-functioning PDD (autism, AS, or PDD without mental retardation) waiting for entry into the Yale Child Study Center's Project on Social Disability. Of these, 60 (55%) were taking psychotropic medications, and 68.8% had taken medication at some point in their lives. Of those taking medication for behavior/emotional problems, over half (53.3%) were taking two or more medications at the same time. The most commonly used medications were antidepressants (32.1%), stimulants (20.2%), and antipsychotics (16.5%). The most common symptoms for which medication was prescribed: anxiety (65%), attention problems (30%), disruptive or self-injurious behavior (43.3%), obsessive-compulsive or repetitive behavior (40%), and depression (28.3%).

Use of psychotropic medications for children in general far outstrips the available scientific evidence of its effectiveness. There is an accumulation of evidence that some medications hold promise for effectiveness with children and adolescents with autism spectrum disorders, but there are no studies looking specifically at children with AS. Extrapolating from the scientific literature is complicated. In terms of general cognitive and adaptive functioning, children with AS are somewhere between typically developing children and the majority of children with autism, so direct extrapolation form either group is not possible.

That said, however, there is good reason to believe that when a child with AS has accompanying emotional symptoms or behavioral disturbance, the addition of medication to a comprehensive intervention package can be quite beneficial. Parents should find a child psychiatrist or pediatric pharmacologist with extensive experience with autism spectrum disorders to partner with in making decisions about the use of medication. Very careful assessment is needed to determine what the target of treatment should be. This can be complicated. For instance, aggressive outbursts might be precipitated by anxiety, by poor impulse control, by problems with emotional regulation, by inflexibility, or by irritability that often accompanies depression in children. The type of medication that is prescribed might vary depending on the presumed underlying cause of the aggression.

Initiating, evaluating, and managing medication for emotional problems is much more time-consuming and complicated than most people realize until they embark on this process. An experienced clinician will gather information from the child, his or her parents, teachers, and possibly other informants, to try to obtain a complete picture of the problem. A trial of medication generally involves a low initial dose, followed by periodic assessment of its effectiveness and dose adjustment as needed. Response to these medications is highly variable from one individual to another. It takes time, sometimes several weeks, to obtain an adequate evaluation of the effects of a particular dose of a particular medication. Changes in medication should occur when all other things are stable (e.g., routine, other interventions, diet) so that one can be reasonably certain that any change in behavior is due to the particular medication in question. The first medication tried might not work, and then the process starts again with another. Some medications require periodic monitoring of blood levels, heart functioning, or other biological systems. Sometimes a medication seems to work well for a period of time and then the effects "go away", necessitating a change to a new medication. This is not meant to discourage parents from trying medication, because we feel that medication can be a very important component of a treatment package. But, parents should be aware upfront of the effort involved, so that they can make informed decisions and do not become discouraged prematurely.

SELECTIVE SEROTONIN REUPTAKE INHIBITORS (*SSRIs*).   In the Yale survey described above (Martin et al., 1999), the most common class of medications prescribed were antidepressants. Most of the antidepressants being used were in the class of medications called SSRIs (selective serotonin-reuptake inhibitors). SSRIs have fewer side effects than other antidepressants, seem to be helpful for a range of mood and behavioral symptoms, and require less medical monitoring than many other available medications. These features make them the preferred medication for many childhood psychiatric disorders. Although new versions of SSRIs appear on the market periodically, the ones most commonly prescribed to children and adolescents are fluvoxamine (Luvox), fluoxetine (Prozac), sertraline (Zoloft), and paroxetine (Paxil).

SSRIs have been shown to be effective in reducing symptoms of anxiety (RUPP Network, 2001), depression (Emslie et al., 1997; Keller et al., 2001), and obsessive compulsive disorder (March et al., 1998; Grados et al., 1999). There is also good evidence that fluvoxamine reduces compulsive behavior and aggression, and increases prosocial behavior in adults with autism spectrum disorders (McDougle, et al., 1996). There is preliminary evidence of the usefulness of fluoxetine in improving global functioning in children with autism spectrum disorders (Cook et al., 1992; DeLong et al., 1998). However, caution is advised, as there is also evidence that SSRIs may be less effective and more likely to cause "behavioral activation" (hyperactivity, agitation, insomnia, aggression) in younger children with autism spectrum disorders (Posey & McDougle, 2000), as well as in children without developmental disorders (Riddle et al., 1992; Scahill et al., 1997). On the other hand, clinical experience suggests that "behavioral activation" might be avoided by starting treatment at a lower dose. There are no definitive studies of the usefulness of SSRIs in children and adolescents specifically within the higher-functioning range of the autism spectrum. Further research is needed to specify whether, and at what dose, these medications might be effective in treating specific symptoms in youth with AS.

OTHER ANTIDEPRESSANTS.   Clomipramine (Anafranil), a mixed serotonin and noreprinephrine uptake inhibitor, has shown mixed results. Two studies (Gordon et al., 1992; Gordon et al., 1993) suggested that clomipramine reduced repetitive behavior and stereotypies in children with autism. Sanchez and colleagues (1996) did not find clomipramine to be effective in a group of younger children. All of these studies did report a fairly high rate of side effects, including moodiness, drowsiness, aggressive behavior, and urinary retention. There are also concerns about increasing seizures and cardiac irregularities. Other antidepressants have either produced unacceptable levels of side effects, or have not been adequately evaluated (Posey & McDougle, 2000).

OTHER ANTI-ANXIETY MEDICATIONS.   Given that anxiety appears to be common in people with AS, there may be a need to find an alternative to SSRIs to treat debilitating anxiety. Unfortunately, there is little science to guide this decision. Buspirone (BuSpar) is a non-benzodiazepine antianxiety medication that has been shown to effectively treat general anxiety and depression, but not obsessive-compulsive disorder, in adults (Riddle et al., 1999). Preliminary trials in children without developmental disorders also suggest that the medication may be helpful in treating anxiety (Wagner, 2001; Riddle, 1999). One pilot study suggested that buspirone may be effective in treating anxiety and irritability in children with autism spectrum disorders (Buitelaar et al., 1998). Because buspirone appears to be free of serious side effects, further investigation of its efficacy in treating anxiety in children with AS would be helpful.

Benzodiazepines (e.g., Xanax, Valium, Ativan) are potent antianxiety medications. They have been studied widely in adults, but very little in children (Riddle et al., 1999). In adults, significant side effects include dependence and withdrawal symptoms, motor incoordination, and tremors (Riddle et al., 1999). These drugs are often used illicitly for their intoxicating effects. For these reasons, they are usually avoided for treating children and adolescents.

PSYCHOSTIMULANTS.   Stimulants such as methylphenidate (Ritalin) and dextroamphetamine (Dexedrine) have been shown to be very effective in treating Attention Deficit Hyperactivity Disorder (ADHD) in children without developmental disorders (for reviews, see Wilens, 2001; American Academy of Pediatrics, 2000, 2001), and in children with mild to moderate cognitive deficits (Aman et al., 1997; Handen et al., 1999). Evidence for their usefulness in children with autism spectrum disorders has been mixed, and there have been no studies investigating its use in children specifically with AS. Clinical anecdotes as well as early case studies and pilot studies (see Posey & McDougle, 2000 for a review) suggested questionable efficacy and an increase in irritability, tantrums, and other side effects in children with autism treated with methylphenidate. However, subsequent studies using small group designs found methylphenidate to be at least modestly helpful in decreasing hyperactivity in children with autism (Birmaher et al., 1988; Quintana et al., 1995).

In the case of stimulants, very careful assessment of the target symptoms is required to determine whether the behaviors of concern are the same as those that are generally treated with stimulants. At times, other symptoms associated with ASD such as inflexibility, lack of attention to social cues, and repetitive motor movements, can mimic ADHD symptoms of inattention and hyperactivity. There is clearly a need for further evaluation of stimulant medication in children with AS. In the meantime, parents should work closely with a professional who has expertise with AS and pediatric pharmacology to make medication decisions.

OTHER TREATMENT FOR HYPERACTIVITY AND INATTENTION. Clonidine (Catapres) is a medication for hypertension that has been used to treat inattention and overactivity in ADHD and Tourette's disorder. Case studies and small clinical trials have suggested it is effective in treating these symptoms in children with autism, although there is evidence that effects "wear off" and that irritability may increase over time (Posey & McDougle, 2000; McDougle, 1997). Concerns about side effects, risk for accidental overdose, and interactions with other drugs have been increasing, and close monitoring is recommended if this medication is used (Posey & McDougle, 2000).

Guanfacine (Tenex) is another hypertension medication that appears to have fewer unwanted side effects. Case studies have suggested its usefulness in treating ADHD in typically developing children and in children with Tourette's disorder (Posey & McDougle, 2000). A well-designed pilot study comparing guanfacine to placebo found that the medication reduced symptoms of inattention and overactivity in children with ADHD and comorbid tic disorder (Scahill et al., 2001). This may be a useful medication for children with AS and inattention/hyperactivity, who do not respond well to stimulants, although there is little scientific evidence to guide clinicians at this time.

Atypical Antipsychotics

Antipsychotic medications were among the first medications evaluated to treat severe behavior problems in autistic adults and children. Several of these medications appeared to be helpful in reducing aggression, overactivity, stereotypies, and withdrawal in autistic children (Posey & McDougle, 2000). Sedation was a common side effect. Of greater concern, was a high frequency of motor problems, including jerkiness during voluntary movements (dyskinesia) and involuntary twitches and motor movements (tardive dyskinesia) (Campbell et al., 1997). Because of these concerns, this medication is generally used only with the most severe behavior problems.

A newer class of antipsychotic medication, called atypical antipsychotics, has promise in treating severe behavioral disturbance in children with developmental disabilities, including autism. Risperidone (Risperdal) was shown to reduce tantrums, aggression, and self-injurious behavior in autistic children over a six month period, without dyskinesia or other severe side effects (RUPP Autism Network, 2002). Weight gain, significant in some cases, was the most common side effect, as well as transient sedation. Olanzapine (Zyprexa) has shown promise in case studies with similar side effects profiles. These medications have not yet been tested for long-term safety and efficacy, however, and they have not been evaluated for use specifically with children with AS. Other atypical antipsychotics, including clozapine (Clozaril) and quetiapine (Seroquel) may increase the risk for seizures or other serious medical conditions (Posey & McDougle, 2000) and need further evaluation of their safety.

Nonstandard Treatments: Helping Parents Be Informed Consumers

Because the cause and underlying biology of autism spectrum disorders are not well understood, it is difficult to know what treatments to pursue. The same principles that apply to the choice of behavioral and medication interventions should be applied to nonstandard treatments as well: careful evaluation of the rationale for the treatment and the evidence of its efficacy; the guidance of an expert in autism spectrum disorders and other consultants if needed; weighing the cost in terms of finances, effort, and potential side effects versus the evidence of beneficial effects. When considering biological interventions such as dietary supplements or medications, it is very important to understand the potential short-term and long-term side effects, as well as potential interactions with other medications. Finally, I would caution parents against diverting their child from interventions that do have evidence of effectiveness to pursue new ones that do not.

Some commonly used interventions simply have not undergone sufficient scientifically rigorous testing to draw conclusions about their usefulness. Following are some of the approaches that have received a lot of attention for treatment of autistic spectrum disorders, but *have not been shown to be effective* in treating the majority of children with autism.

Auditory integration training is an approach in which the child listens to a variety of sounds with the goal of improving language comprehension. Advocates of this method suggest that it helps people with autism receive more balanced sensory input from their environment. When tested using rigorous scientific procedures, the method was shown to be no more effective than listening to music (Bettison, 1996; Zollweg et al., 1997; Dawson & Watling, 2000). The American Academy of Pediatrics (2001) has recommended against the use of auditory integration training.

Dietary interventions are based on the idea that food allergies cause symptoms of autism. Proponents of this approach argue that removing the allergy-causing food from the child's diet can relieve these symptoms. Although a nutritious, well-balanced diet is important for the general health of children with PDDs, there is currently no scientifically based evidence that food allergies are related to symptoms in the majority of persons with autism or other PDDs. Additionally, some children on special "elimination" diets have shown signs of significant malnutrition related to the degree of restriction the diet imposes on other essential nutrients. Therefore, it is especially crucial that a child's nutritional status be monitored carefully if a special diet is tried.

One of the more widely known dietary interventions for autism is the *gluten-free, casein-free diet*. This treatment is based on the theory that gluten and casein produce substances that can have a toxic effect on the brain, leading to autistic symptoms. It has been suggested that gastrointestinal problems sometimes experienced by children with autism make the digestive tract "leaky" enough to allow gluten and casein to seep through the intestinal wall into the blood stream, where they are carried to the brain. Eliminating gluten and casein from the diet would, theoretically, prevent their affecting the brain. Another approach, called *enzyme therapy*, would add special enzymes to the diet to remove the toxic substances from the digestive tract. Neither of these approaches has been tested in rigorous scientific studies (American Academy of Pediatrics, 2001), and the effect on nutritional status of restricting diets in this way has not been documented.

Vitamin B6, taken with magnesium, has been explored as a way to stimulate brain activity. Because vitamin B6 plays an important role in creating enzymes needed by the brain, some experts predict that large doses might foster greater brain activity in people with autism. However, clinical studies of the vitamin have been difficult to interpret due to methodological problems (Pfeiffer et al., 1995; American Academy of Pediatrics, 2001). Low doses of vitamins probably pose little risk of harm, but higher doses can be toxic. Parents should always discuss the risks of administering vitamin or nutritional supplements with a physician before embarking on such a treatment.

Secretin is a hormone commonly given in tests to diagnosis gastrointestinal problems. A natural form of secretin is derived from pigs, and a synthetic form has also been produced. Interest in secretin as a treatment for autism arose following the publication of reports of a child whose autism symptoms improved after a single dose of secretin. Since then, however, several carefully conducted studies of persons with autism have reported not finding any significant benefits from secretin when given in its porcine or synthetic form, or with single or multiple doses (Unis, A.S., Munson, J.A., Rogers, S.J. et al., 2002). Additionally there have been concerns raised about the possibility of allergic reactions to repeated doses of secretin. The American Academy of Pediatrics (2001) concluded that there was no evidence to justify the use of secretin infusion treatment in children with autism spectrum disorders.

Lack of evidence for a particular treatment is not the same thing as evidence against its usefulness. Parents should be informed and should obtain professional assistance in understanding the theoretical underpinnings of an emerging, new treatment, the state of the scientific evidence available, and the costs/risks involved in the treatment. Information about other nonstandard treatments can be found in practice parameters and guidelines published in professional journals (American Academy of Child and Adolescent Psychiatry, 1999; Filipek et al., 2000; American Academy of Pediatrics, 2001).

Summary

There is little scientific evidence to guide families and caregivers in choosing treatment and support strategies for children with AS. We hope that the increasing awareness of the syndrome will lead to more and better research. In the meantime, there are strategies available with theoretical and clinical support for their usefulness, (and preliminary evidence in some cases) which can alleviate strain and symptoms when they occur and promote optimal adaptive functioning. Children and adolescents with a diagnosis of AS require a carefully measured, multi-modal method of intervention that includes psychoeducation, behavioral and cognitive-behavioral strategies, and, often, medication treatments and monitoring. This chapter presents a parent-professional team approach to determining when there is a need for intervention, and how to choose the most appropriate interventions for the needs of a particular child and his or her family.

APPENDIX A. Functional Analysis

Assess Level of Emotional Arousal

This first step helps to identify the antecedents to emotional escalation and behavioral decompensation. These antecedents are unique to each individual. What are the triggering events? What are the early warning signs of emotional escalation? What are the early warning signs of behavioral decompensation? What happens if emotions continue to escalate and behavior continues to decompensate? The goal is to create a clear description of these events from inception to full escalation, in order to identify windows of opportunity for intervention.

For the AS child, often these are the situations/events that tax his or her ability to be flexible or incorporate requests to do something differently. The seemingly impossible demand, often accompanied with perceived rejection, leads to overwhelming internal arousal. Therefore, identifying the triggering event provides the opportunity to intervene and prevent decompensation or acting out in reaction to frustration. For example, a triggering event for "Alex" (not his real name) was receiving critical feedback about his behavior from his teacher. His internal early warning signs included feeling frustrated ("butterflies" in his stomach, sweaty palms, shallow breathing). Externally, he became fidgety, was off-task, and began to use nonsequitors. If this process continued uninterrupted, "Alex" would escalate to loud arguing, refusal to comply, pacing about the room, and sometimes running out of the classroom.

Alex's teacher learned to provide corrective feedback in a less critical manner, helped "Alex" to identify when to stop and separate from a frustrating situation, so that he could have a 10–minute "cooling-off" period away from the frustrating situation. Sometimes "Alex" would engage in some outdoor physical activity, such as shooting baskets, or walking, to appropriately dispel the built-up energy.

After the antecedents to Emotional Arousal have been identified, the next step is to assess level of skill in three areas: Behavioral, Cognitive, and Self-Control. Through this assessment process, areas of strength and weakness will be discerned.

Behavioral Difficulties

APPROPRIATE SOCIAL SKILLS? There are three questions that must be answered in this section:

1. Does the AS child have the appropriate social skills that are needed to interact in an acceptable social manner?

2. Has the student been able to pick up social cues throughout his/her life to learn socially acceptable behavior?
3. Does s/he have the cognitive and language processing abilities to assimilate the knowledge of socially acceptable behavior?

Given that social skills weakness is one of the primary features of AS, the child with AS invariably lacks age-appropriate social skills to some degree. One will need to determine what types of situations are causing difficulty, and specifically which skills are not yet developed. One of the many contributing factors to this deficit is the inability to "read" nonverbal social cues. However, most AS children do have a desire to develop "friendships", although their concept of a friend is qualitatively different than the generally accepted concept of "friendship." The challenge is how to go about helping them develop these skills. To accomplish this, we need to know the nature of their cognitive and language processing abilities.

The AS child typically does possess the cognitive intelligence to learn these skills. However, as will be identified in a later section, cognitive rigidity and impaired ability to take on the perspective of others significantly interferes with learning socially acceptable behaviors.

The way in which information is presented for learning is another consideration. Many AS children learn more efficiently if information is presented to them through the visual medium: pictures and icons. They are less efficient at learning when information is presented in a primarily auditory format. The distinction between auditory and visual material is an important distinction of which to be aware: not all visual material is purely visual. For example, the printed word (e.g. textbooks) is processed not only through the visual centers of the brain, but also the speech centers. And the speech center is an area of weakness. Pictures and icons are more purely visually processed forms of information.

Learning is further enhanced when the other sensory modalities (touch, taste, smell) are also incorporated. Language processing skills are also impaired in the AS youngster, particularly in the area of language pragmatics – the practical application of language. A thorough assessment of language pragmatics should be part of the pre-intervention assessment process. The Learning Clinic's Pragmatic Skills Survey (*Ducharme, 1992*) is an effective tool for identifying level of language skill development, and will be discussed later.

Because of this level of social skill impairment, the AS child will need social skills training. Based on the foregoing, the social skills training should be multi-sensory, with an emphasis on the visual medium, e.g., videotaped role-plays of social scenarios, with video feedback. Role-plays also should be designed to provide practice at taking on another's perspective, and cognitive flexibility, e.g., identifying multiple solutions to social dilemmas, and incorporating feedback.

The social skill role-plays should also include training in the specific areas of pragmatic skill deficits identified through the Pragmatic Skills Survey.

Level of Response-Contingent Reinforcement?

This section assesses whether or not a student's behavior can be modified by contingency management, and what type of reinforcements are effective.

The questions to be answered in this section include:

1. What is the student's level of response to reinforcement contingencies?
2. Does the environment reinforce the correct targeted behavior?
3. If not, what behavior does it reinforce?

Common motivators for people in general include reinforcements that have a social component. For example, providing a student an opportunity to participate in an activity with a friend is generally an effective motivator. However, opportunities for social interaction are not motivating for an AS child. What is generally more effective is to use the Premack Principal: opportunity to participate in a preferred activity is contingent upon first participating in a nonpreferred activity. This is an example of how capitalize upon an area of strength to develop what is lacking.

To identify an effective motivator for an AS youngster, you must first identify the student's areas of interest. For example, "Alex" likes trains and wrestling: reading about the history, design and construction of trains, riding trains, learning about train schedules, watching wrestling videos, reading wrestling magazines, and attending wrestling events. To motivate "Alex" to develop social skills, he is required to participate in social interactions before he can participate in one of his preferred activities. For example, for one hour of social interaction, "Alex" earns 20 minutes time to read one of his train or wrestling books.

Cognitive Functioning

COGNITIVE DISTORTIONS.   The goal of this section is to assess the degree to which a student can accurately process the available information in his environment. The questions to be answered include:

1. Does the student have the ability to reflect and evaluate his/her behavior?
2. Does the student have maladaptive or dysfunctional thinking patterns?
3. Or, do they perceive situations, but are unable to evaluate the situation with an accurate perspective?

The AS child has multiple deficits which interfere with the ability to accurately process information: impaired perspective-taking, difficulty reading nonverbal cues, literal interpretation of information, and impaired comprehension of meaning.

The impaired ability to take on the perspective of another person significantly contributes to difficulties in this area. For example, one hot summer day, "Alex" went to the refrigerator to get some ice for his water glass. When he found the ice tray empty, he wailed, "Why did they do this to me? They knew I would be coming in for some ice, and deliberately used it all up so I wouldn't have any!" No amount of consolation or explanation could convince "Alex" that no one did this to him deliberately.

The difficulty "reading" nonverbal cues also leads to distortion of information. For example, while talking at length with a group of peers about his interest in trains, "Alex" failed to notice that the group of peers was rapidly dwindling. Peers had regrouped into other conversational groups. Nor did he respond to the yawns, eye gaze directed elsewhere in the room, and other body language the conveyed loss of interest. "Alex" continued to talk about his trains until the last person simply walked away. "Alex's" recount of this interaction was that he had many friends who were interested in what he had to say about trains.

The tendency toward literal interpretation of information also leads to misinformation. The use of colloquialisms, metaphors, and analogies are generally lost on the AS child. They tend to interpret information literally. For example, "Alex" was speaking with a teacher one day who stated that she was so busy lately that she thought she might meet herself coming around the corner. "Alex" immediately corrected her and stated, "That's impossible! You can't meet yourself!"

AS students also sometimes fail to comprehend the meaning of words. At the same time, these students tend not to ask for clarification. Typically, they want to fit in, and therefore feign comprehension. Unless their understanding is confronted, this misunderstanding of intended meaning goes undetected. For example, "Alex" was participating in a social skills group, and was instructed to view a videotape of their role-play and identify the use of "negotiating", "assertiveness", and use of "eye contact." His accuracy score was 53.3 %. After his understanding of the target skills was confronted, he revealed that he did not understand what these words meant. "Alex" was rehearsed on the meaning of the words, and provided with peer demonstration of them. When "Alex" rated the video a second time, his accuracy score was 100%.

Problem-Solving Deficit?

If there is a problem with accurate perception or processing of information, then problem-solving skills will be similarly impacted. The questions to be answered in this section include:

1. Does the student have the problem-solving and organizational skills needed to solve problems?
2. Can the student accurately read context cues and adjust his/her behavior accordingly?
3. Does the student have the ability to identify ineffective strategies?
4. Does the student have the ability to effectively apply the correct strategy?

For the AS child, problem-solving skills are often poor. In addition to having accurate information, effective problem-solving requires good executive function skills and a good working memory. Generally, executive function skills (organizing, planning, sequencing) are poor. When left to his own resources, the AS student does not effectively organize and sequence information. They fail to anticipate events and plan for contingencies.

Good problem-solving skills are also dependent upon the ability to hold a lot of information in working memory, to remember previously learned "rules", then apply those rules to the stored information, and manipulate that information to arrive at the correct solution.

These skill are all lacking in the AS child. "Alex" has repeatedly had difficulty living within a budget, and often is overdrawn on his bank accounts. "Alex" had been given a limit of $20 withdrawals from his ATM account, and these withdrawals could be done only under two conditions: with prior parent approval, or in case of an emergency. One month his parent noted frequent unauthorized ATM withdrawals, occurring every 2–3 days. "Alex" was confronted on his frequent withdrawals from his ATM account. He insisted that he was not aware that he had used the ATM so frequently. He also believed he had done nothing wrong because he only used the ATM for "emergencies." He never kept the ATM receipts, and his definition of an emergency included buying food when he was hungry, purchasing a present for a family member's birthday, paying for entertainment expenses to occupy his time, etc.

Modifying your behavior in response to the needs to others requires that you first be able to "read" the contextual cues which provide the information about the needs of others. Because AS children are generally poor at reading these nonverbal, contextual cues, they fail to take in vital information which would inform them about the needs of others. From their perspective, they have made the correct behavioral choice based on the information which they have processed. For example, "Alex" had parked his car in a row of cars. As he was backing out, he heard a muffled "thump". He continued to back out of the parking space, then got out and checked his car. He did not see any damage to his car, so he assumed the "thump" sound had nothing to do with him or his car. It did not occur to him to check for damage to the other person's car. As he was pulling away, he saw a car bumper lying in the parking lot, but again he assumed it had nothing to do with him, as he had already checked his car. Later that night, the police came to his home. They informed him that as he pulled out of the parking space, three people witnessed him pulling the bumper off one car, and sideswiping two other cars. The three witnesses had chased after "Alex's" car, waving their arms to signal him to stop, but he kept driving off.

"Alex" was adamant that he did not see the people chasing after him. He was also insistent that he had done nothing wrong because he had checked his car and did not see anything wrong with it. Obviously, "Alex" failed to process multiple, vital contextual cues. Based on the information which he processed, he concluded that he could not have done that of which he was accused.

Another common problem for "Alex" is irritating his peers by intruding on their conversations. Typically when "Alex" wants to share a story with others he will walk up to a group of peers and begin talking, regardless of any ongoing conversations. "Alex" fails to take notice of the activities and conversations which are already in progress. He does not know how to wait for an opportune moment to enter a conversation.

SELF-CONTROL. This section of the Functional Analysis assesses whether or not the student has developed an internal locus of control. This includes the ability to remember previously stated rules, and to use those rules to guide behavior. The questions to be answered in this section include:

1. Does the student have impulse control?
2. Does the student remember previously stated rules, directions, and rehearsal?
3. Is the student able to learn to self-regulate?
4. Is the student able to perform skills with cues?
5. Is the student able to perform appropriate learned skills without prompt from cues?

The AS child generally makes an effort to follow the rules – as he understands them. The challenge is to help the student learn the rules and internalize them. The difference between the AS student and an oppositional-defiant student is volition. The oppositional student will planfully disobey the rules, whereas the AS student does so because he either misunderstood the application of the rule, or acted impulsively. Poor attention and concentration and impulsivity are not uncommon due to executive function deficits.

With frequent rehearsals and cueing, the AS student can learn to self-regulate. However, a rule learned in one setting will not necessarily be applied in a similar setting. This difficulty has to do with the misreading of contextual cues. If a few salient contextual cues change from one environment to another, the AS student is likely to perceive the similar setting/situation as entirely different.

To facilitate consistent application of a rule, it's important to teach the AS student to recognize and use environmental cues that are generally available in multiple settings. For example, a cue that elicits the behavior in the school setting, should also be a cue that is available at home, at work, in the community, etc. For example, if the AS student is old enough to safely self-administer his/her own medication, a wrist alarm watch can be used to signal times of administration. The wrist alarm becomes the medication cue that is present in all settings. The traffic light signals and road signs are other examples of cues that are available in multiple settings.

As the AS student is learning the cues to guide behavior, s/he must also learn to self-monitor progress, self-evaluate, self-reinforce, and self-instruct. Self-monitoring is best accomplished through concrete, written recordings of progress. A calendar can be used to record frequency counts of successful results. Self-evaluation includes modifying behavior as needed. Reinforcement of success is vital to encourage perseverance in developing a skill. Since other people are not always going to be available to provide that reinforcement, it is essential to teach the AS student how to self-reinforce. Examples of self-reinforcement include treating oneself to a favorite meal, saving up for and buying a special item, providing verbal praise, etc.

Self-instruction is used as a means to sequentially guide oneself through the steps of the task. Because AS children do not engage in subvocal speech to guide behavior, it's important to teach them to self-instruct out loud, but at a low volume. Self-instruction helps to focus attention on the steps of the task, incorporating needed modifications, and completing it.

Problem Identification Leads to Intervention Strategy

Below is the functional analysis presented in schematic form. It demonstrates how the identification of a skills deficit or otherwise locating a source of difficulty leads directly to the choice of intervention strategy.

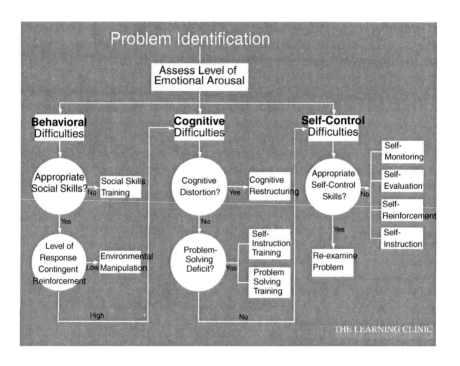

APPENDIX B. The Learning Clinic Pragmatic Skills
Survey Model

Pragmatic language refers to the practical use of language, and includes both verbal and nonverbal communication. It involves what it said, why it is said, and when to use certain forms of speech. Both the use and understanding of the complexities of language are challenges for AS students. Assessment of these skills, therefore, is vital to identifying the level of skill development and areas for intervention. The Learning Clinic Pragmatic Skills Survey (DuCharme, 1992) is an assessment tool designed to describe the level of social communication skills. The survey results identify areas of strength, and areas of weakness, that will require intervention and skill-building.

The Pragmatic Skills Survey assesses four categories of communication: topic, purpose, abstraction, and visual/gestural cues. The survey results provide a functional description of the student's communication skills with adults, with peers, and in various settings. A Likert scale (0–5) is used to rate each of the 65 items on the survey. A score of 0 = skill absent, and a score of 5 = age-appropriate development of the skill and ability to use it appropriately in all settings. A score of 0–2 indicates the need for intervention, while a rating of 3 would suggest the need for further observation to determine if intervention is needed. Average subtotal scores are calculated for each category, as well as an overall average for all 65 items.

The Pragmatic Skills Survey was administered to a group of AS youngsters at The Learning Clinic. These group average scores for peer to peer interactions (in a school setting) are presented below.

Topic

The first category, Topic, is defined as the "subject" of the communication. To assess the ability to appropriately choose a topic, there are several areas to evaluate: 1) establishing a conversation; 2) maintaining a conversation; 3) content of the topic; 4) changing topics appropriately; 5) revising messages to fit changes in topic; 6) modifying messages to repair breakdown in communication; and 7) appropriately terminating a conversation.

ESTABLISHES CONVERSATION. In assessing this area, we want to know if the student can appropriately *establish* a conversation. To appropriately establish a conversation one has to be able to *select* and *introduce* a topic. Is the AS student able to chose from an array of topics and decide upon one? Does s/he know how to initiate the presentation of the information to others?

Typically, AS students tend to choose either immature topics of conversation, or a topic in which others have very little interest. When introducing a topic, they fail to attend to social cues which would inform them of the appropriate time for entering into a conversation. Average score for topic selection was 1.92 and 1.69 for introduction of a topic.

Maintains Conversation

We also need to assess the ability to appropriately *maintain a conversation*. This includes how long one speaks (the *duration* of the topic), and appropriate *turn-taking*. Is the AS student "long-winded" when speaking? Does s/he wait for a pause in the conversation before speaking, or does s/he interrupt others? Does s/he monopolize the conversation, or give others "space" to speak?

The ability to maintain a conversation decreased as the duration increased. For 1 minute the average score was 2.92. At 15 minutes, the average score decreased to 0.85. Appropriate turn-taking skills averaged 2.0. Typically, AS students either interrupt others, or fail to participate in the conversation unless prompted to do so.

CONTENT OF TOPIC.   Content of topic is assessed in terms of *accuracy*, *logic*, *relevance*, and *conciseness*. Accuracy: is the information which is being presented accurate, or is it distorted? Logic: is the AS student able to speak in a logical manner? Is the information reasonable, and does it represent sound judgment? Does one thought logically follow another without the introduction of non-relevant data, themes or questions? Relevance: is the information relevant to the people with whom s/he is speaking and to the setting in which it occurs? Conciseness: refers to the under or over-elaboration of information, or perseveration. Is the student able to present information in an appropriately concise manner? Can s/he be succinct? Perseveration refers to the student's inability to shift ideas. It is a restricted, limiting scope within the boundaries of the topics.

When providing information, the AS student ranges from distorted to very accurate. Their average score was 2.69 for accuracy. Logic and relevance averaged 2.15 each, while conciseness was 1.92. In general, AS students tend to be long-winded and introduce nonrelevant data because of their circumscribed interest in the topic. They also fail to read social cues which would inform them of the waning interest of their "audience" and the need to allow others time to speak.

CHANGES TOPIC APPROPRIATELY.   Can the AS student change the topic of conversation to coincide with shifts in the conversation? Can s/he incorporate verbal and nonverbal cues to know when a change in topic is appropriate? Does s/he demonstrate cognitive flexibility to shift from one topic to another? Are changes in topic preceded by appropriate introduction of the new topic and transitional statements?

It is not unusual for the AS student to miss the shifts on the conversation, and to rigidly continue speaking on their topic of interest. Conversations can also seem "disconnected" because of the failure of the AS student to use transitional statements to connect one topic to another. Average score for this skill was 1.69.

REVISES MESSAGE TO FIT CHANGE IN TOPIC.   When new information is received, can the AS student revise messages within the flow of reciprocal conversation? Or does s/he rigidly adhere to previously formed concepts and opinions, failing to incorporate the new information?

Cognitive rigidity, restricted range of interest, and failure to read the social cues contributes to the difficulty in this area. For example, when "Alex" is given information that contradicts his firmly held beliefs about his favorite sports team scoring record, he dismisses the information, and continues to state his belief. Average score was 1.46.

MODIFIES MESSAGE TO REPAIR BREAKDOWN IN COMMUNICATION.   When the AS student perceives that the person intended to receive the message did not understand it, can s/he modify the message? Can s/he adjust the message so that it is better understood?

Average score for this skill was 1.46. AS students in general have great difficulty rephrasing messages to make themselves better understood. For example, when "Alex" was informed by a peer that he did not understand what he had said, "Alex" simply repeated himself, speaking more slowly and with more emphasis the second time.

TERMINATES CONVERSATION APPROPRIATELY.   Does the AS student use appropriate closing statements? Or does s/he just walk away, or start another activity when done speaking?

The tendency of AS students is to stop speaking (or walk away) when they are done speaking, with no closing statements. Average score was 1.69

Purpose

Purpose of the conversation is the second category of the survey. The purpose is the inferred "why" behind the communication. A message may be delivered with varying degrees of directness, politeness, and clarity. Purpose has five sub-components, with elaboration for each subcomponent.

REQUESTING/ASKING.   Requesting/asking can be done with the "Who-When-What-Why-How" interrogatives, or by using inflection, e.g., upward tone at the end of a sentence. When assessing the AS student's ability to appropriately use requests or questions, there are several qualities of inquiry to evaluate. For example, can the AS students ask questions that are in the form of an either/or choice? Do they inquire about another's emotions, sensations, or intents? Can they ask product questions – questions that require a response that involves a product, such as information? For example, "What kind of video games do you own?

Another type of question is the process question. Does the AS student ask questions that elicit information about a process/sequence of steps? For example, "Okay, after I get home from school, what do I have to do before I can watch TV?" Or, "After I vacuum and dust my room, what do I do next?"

Does the AS student ask questions that request an action? For example, "Could you please make spaghetti and meatballs for dinner tonight?" And, can they ask permission for an action or object? For example, "Can I ride your bike for awhile?"

Do they ask for clarification of a prior remark? Or do they feign understanding and avoid asking for clarification? Can they ask questions which suggest an action? For example, "Don't you agree that we should go camping before the weather gets too cold?

Scores for requesting/asking ranged from 1.54 to 2.23. The inability to predict what others are thinking or feeling contributed to the low score in this section: asking about another's emotions (1.54); asking questions that suggest an action (1.61); asking for clarification of a prior remark (1.85). They were more skilled at asking product questions (2.23).

INFORMING.   Informing refers to the use of statements to convey specific information. It can be a relevant response to a question.

Informing can take several forms. For example, does the AS student use statements to explain, describe, or identify things? Do they express personal judgments, opinions, attitudes, agreements, or disagreements? Do they use statements to express beliefs about other's abilities? Do they inform others of their choices, answer questions, or indicate their compliance?

Expressing their belief about another's abilities was the greatest area of difficulty in this category (1.23). As above, their difficulty predicting what others think or feel impairs skill in this area. They were more skilled at answering choice questions (2.08), and explaining/describing (2.08).

Regulating

Regulating pertains to the use of statements that are intended to control another's behavior, to get one's attention, negotiate, or influence actions. There are many ways in which we can attempt to regulate others. This includes using warnings or reminders when appropriate. Delineating personal claims is another form of regulating. For example, making a statement that identifies a personal claim/right to property, privilege, etc.: "That's my bicycle!" or "It's my turn next."

Other forms of regulating are labeling the speaker who gets the next turn, or using persuasion appropriately. When we offer assistance, or object to another's behavior/demand, or negate another's statement/behavior we are attempting to regulate. And lastly, attempting to delay or speed-up the actions of oneself or others is also a form of regulating.

In general, scores for regulating were low. The highest score in this section was 2.15 for objecting to another's behavior. Students were least skilled at attempting to speed-up or delay the actions of self or others (1.39). Low average scores were also obtained for appropriate use of persuasion, reminders and warnings (average score for each was 1.46).

EXPRESSING (RECEPTIVE/EXPRESSIVE).   Expressing includes both the *use* of expressive statements, and the *understanding* of others' use of the same. Expressing is a type of language that uses statements to describe a person's emotions, sensations, intents, beliefs, or that label or elicit emotions in others. This includes identifying one's own emotions, e.g., "That hurts," or other-directed comments, e.g., "You look happy." Expressing can also predict, e.g., "If I draw a nice picture, my father will be proud of me."

There are many ways to use expressive statements. For example, does the AS student use statements to express the emotions, sensations, intents of himself/herself? And can s/he do the same for others? Does s/he tell jokes? Does s/he understand and respond appropriately to others' jokes? Does she apologize, congratulate, or exclaim appropriately?

Can the AS student use teasing, annoying or provoking of others in a playful, good-natured manner? Does s/he understand and respond appropriately when s/he is the target of playful, good-natured teasing? Is the volume of his/her voice appropriate to the setting and situation? Is his/her tone of voice consistent with the situation and intent?

Using and understanding teasing were the areas of greatest difficulty in this section (1.39 and 1.46 respectively). Similarly, telling and responding appropriately to jokes were areas of weakness (1.54 and 1.77 respectively). The AS student tends to process information concretely. The ability to use and understand teasing and joking requires the ability to abstract—to understand the irony of placing the message in another context. Higher scores were achieved for apologizing (2.15), using appropriate volume (2.15) and congratulating (2.01).

RITUALIZING.   Ritualizing refers to a type of social communication that involves an "automatic" element in the response, e.g., the use of good manners and common social amenities. A person may excuse themselves when they sneeze, step in front of another, burp, interrupt a conversation, etc.

Ritualizing can also refer to the use of automatic social exchanges with a specific context—audience. For example, the waitress who approaches a table of patrons and asks, "May I take your order?" Or the sales clerk who asks, "May I help you?" Or the emcee who steps up to the microphone and says, "Good afternoon ladies and gentlemen."

The highest scores in this section were for "politeness" and general good manners (1.85). However, adjusting their greetings to fit the context/audience was more difficult (1.69). In general, the AS student demonstrates a desire to please, and with skill training, can learn the social amenities. However, adjusting these skills to fit changes in context and audience is more difficult because of the difficulty reading the social cues.

ABSTRACTION.   Abstraction pertains to a type of message that is communicated by language that is not concrete. An abstract message requires inference and it usually relates to mood, tone, audience, and event. Nonverbal cues are relied upon more heavily for interpretation than the statement itself. The student's intent is to communicate a relationship, image, or emotion that cannot be conveyed in direct terms. "Hints" need to be combined to sum up the message.

To assess the AS student's use of abstraction, we want to know can s/he use sarcasm appropriately? Does s/he understand and respond appropriately to sarcasm? Can s/he use idioms and figurative language appropriately? Does s/he understand and respond appropriately to idioms and figurative language?

Does the AS student use indirect messages? This involves the use of nonverbal communication to convey the message. For example, a student notices a group of peers gathered around another peer who is sharing a bag of chips. He stands nearby, wide-eyed, licking his lips, and inquires, "Are those good?" The indirect message, "Can I have some chips?" is indirectly communicated by the close proximity, wide-eyes, and lip-licking behaviors.

We also need to assess the ability of the AS student to understand and respond appropriately when others use indirect communication.

This is the weakest category for AS youngsters with scores ranging from 1.08–1.77. As with the skills of teasing and joking, AS students in general do not do well with abstractions because of their tendency to process information concretely.

VISUAL/GESTURAL CUES.   Visual/gestural cues refer to nonverbal means of communicating attitudes, moods, or affective states in general. Eye contact, posture, facial expression, proximity, and body movements are elements of visual/gestural cues. This sections assesses not only the use of visual/gestural cues, but also the ability to the AS student to appropriately respond to others' use of these cues.

EYE CONTACT. Eye contact can be initiated, sustained, diverted, or avoided. Does the AS student use eye contact appropriate to the situation? Or does s/he tend to avoid eye contact, or use it inconsistently?

Does the AS student respond appropriately to other's eye contact?

Average score for use of eye contact was 1.85, while responding appropriately to eye contact was 1.69. In general, use of this skill tends to be awkward and inconsistent. With social skill training, AS students tend to improve in their appropriate use of eye contact.

GESTURES/BODY POSTURE. Body language (posture) can be consistent with the message and enhance it, or inconsistent and thereby confuse the message. For example, arms folded, sideway stance, shifting position, unrelated and/or competing body movements in relation to the message are observable indices of socially appropriate communication, or interfering behaviors. Does the AS student use gestures and body posture appropriate to the person, setting, communication?

Does the AS student accurately "read" others' use of body language? Does s/he respond appropriately?

FACIAL EXPRESSION. Facial expression such as a frown or smile are nonverbal forms of communication. Does the AS student use facial expressions? Are these facial expressions consistent with their verbal message, inconsistent, or is there an absence of facial expression? Is the use of facial expression appropriate for the setting?

Does the AS student accurately "read" and respond to others' use of facial expressions?

In general, the use of, and ability to "read" facial gestures were similarly impaired. Average scores for use of facial expressions was 1.85, while response to others' use of facial expressions was 1.92.

The ability to appropriately "read" and respond to others' use of body language was somewhat better than the ability to use the same. The average score for use of appropriate body language was 1.61, while the ability to appropriately read and respond to the same in others was 1.92.

Overall, the AS student's use of facial expression and body gestures tends to be awkward. For example, when "Alex" was learning about the appropriate use of nonverbal communication, he participated in the creation of a chart which listed common body language and facial expressions associated with specific emotions. When participating in role-plays to practice these skills, he would first glance at the chart, to determine which facial and body language expressions he should be using. The end product, although accurate, was awkward in appearance. Although his skill level has improved over time, it continues to have an awkward appearance.

PROXIMITY/DISTANCE.   Proximity refers to the distance one stands from another. Is the AS student aware of others' personal space, and does s/he maintain a distance of at least an arm's length from others? Do they invade others' personal space by standing too close, or bumping into others as they pass by?

When others adjust their distance from the AS student, does s/he respond appropriately? For example, if another person increases his distance from the AS student, does s/he move closer? Or, does s/he remain standing where they are to demonstrate an understanding that the other person wants more personal space between them?

Does the AS student demonstrate differential use of personal space with close friends and family versus casual acquaintances and strangers? Do they adjust their use of personal space for different settings? For example, do they demonstrate an understanding that personal space for friends and family members is different in a public versus a private setting?

The average score for use (1.92) and response (2.07) to proximity was about the same. This is an area where the AS youngster needs ongoing skill training.

PHYSICAL CONTACT.   Physical contact refers to the use of touch as a means of communication, and to influence the behavior of others. Does the AS student demonstrate an understanding and use of touch to facilitate communication? Do they use touch in an appropriate way? Are they aware of and use common forms of physical contact to communicate with others. For example, does s/he use "high fives" with peers to compliment them or to affirm an agreement? When s/he wants someone's attention does s/he tap them lightly on the arm to get their attention? Is s/he aware of the need to avoid physical contact with another's private body parts?

When another person touches the AS student, how does s/he respond? Is the response appropriate to the person and to the context?

As with proximity, the AS student requires ongoing skill training in the appropriate use and response to physical contact. The average score for appropriate use of physical contact was 0.92, while the average score for responding appropriately to physical contact was 1.00. These scores are consistent with the overall negative response of AS youngsters to touch.

References

Aman, M.D., Kern, R.A., Osborne, P., Tumuluru, R., Rojahn, J., Del Medico, V. (1997). Fenfluramine and methylphenidate in children with mental retardation and borderline IQ: Clinical effects. *American Journal on Mental Retardation, 101*(5), 521–534.

American Academy of Child and Adolescent Psychiatry (1999). Practice parameters for the assessment and treatment of children, adolescents, and adults with autism and other pervasive developmental disorders. *Journal of the American Academy of Child and Adolescent Psychiatry, 38,* 32S–54S.

American Academy of Pediatrics (2000). Clinical practice guideline: diagnosis and evaluation of the child with attention-deficit/hyperactivity disorder. *Pediatrics, 105*(5), 1158–1170.

American Academy of Pediatrics (2001). Clinical practice guideline: treatment of the school-aged child with attention-deficit/hyperactivity disorder. *Pediatrics, 108*(4), 1033–1044.

American Academy of Pediatrics (2001). Technical report: The pedatrician's role in the diagnosis and management of autistic spectrum disorder in children. *Pediatrics, 107,* 1–18.

Baker, M.J., Koegel, R.L., Koegel, L.K. (1998). Increasing the social behavior of young children with autism using their obsessive behaviors. *Journal of the Association for Persons with Severe Handicaps, 23*(4), 300–308.

Bettison, S. (1996). The long-term effects of auditory training on children with autism. *Journal of Autism and Developmental Disorders, 26,* 361–374.

Birmaher, B., Quintana, H., Greenhill, L.L. (1988). Methylphenidate treatment of hyperactive autistic children. *Journal of the American Academy of Child and Adolescent Psychiatry, 27,* 248–251.

Buitelaar, J.K., Van der Gaag, R.J., Van der Hoeven, J. (1998). Buspirone in the management of anxiety and irritability in children with pervasive developmental disorders: results of an open-label study. *Journal of Clinical Psychiatry, 59,* 56–59.

Campbell, M., Armenteros, J.L., Malone, R.P., Adams, P.B., Eisenberg, Z.W. (1997). Neuroleptic-related dyskinesias in autistic children: a prospective, longitudinal study. *Journal of the American Academy of Child and Adolescent Psychiatry, 36,* 835–843.

Charlop, M.H., Milstein, J.P. (1989). Teaching autistic children conversational speech using video modeling. *Journal of Applied Behavioral Analysis, 22,* 275–285.

Cook, E.H., Rowlett, R., Jaselskis, C., Leventhal, B.L. (1992). Fluoxetine treatment of children and adults with autistic disorder and mental retardation. *Journal of the American Academy of Child and Adolescent Psychiatry, 31,* 739–745.

Dawson, G., Osterling, J. (1997). Early intervention in autism. In M. Guralnick (Ed.), *The Effectiveness of Early Intervention: Second Generation Research* (pp. 307–326). Baltimore, MD: Brookes.

Dawson, G., Watling, R. (2000). Interventions to facilitate auditory, visual, and motor integration in autism: A review of the evidence. *Journal of Autism and Developmental Disorders, 30,* 415–421.

DeLong, G.R., Teague, L.A., McSwain-Kamran, M. (1998). Effects of fluoxetine treatment in young children with idiopathic autism. *Developmental Medicine and Child Neurology, 40,* 551–562.

DuCharme, R.W. (1992). The Learning Clinic Pragmatic Skills Survey.

DuCharme, R. (in press). Evidence-Based Instruction for children with Asperger Syndrome. In R. DuCharme & T.P. Gullotta (Eds.). Asperger Syndrome: A Handbook for Professionals and Families. NY: Kluwer Academic/Plenum Publishers.

Dugan, E.P., Kamps, D.M., Leonard, B.R., Watkins, N., Rheinberger, A., Stackhaus, J. (1995). Effects of cooperative learning groups during social studies for students with autism and fourth-grade peers. *Journal of Applied Behavior Analysis, 28,* 175–188.

Dunlap, G., Fox, L. (1999). A demonstration of behavioral support for young children with autism. *Journal of Positive Behavioral Interventions, 2,* 77–87.

Dunlap, G., Fox, L. (2001). Early intervention and serious problem behaviors: A comprehensive approach. In Koegel, L.K., Koegel, R.L., Dunlap G. (Eds.), *Positive Behavioral*

Support: Including People with Difficult Behavior in the Community (pp. 3–30). Baltimore, MD: Brookes Publishing.

Emslie, G.J., Rush, A.J., Weinberg, W.A., Kowatch, R.A., Hughes, C.W., Carmody, T., et al. (1997). A double-blind, randomized, placebo-controlled trial of fluoxetine in children and adolescents with depression. *Archives of General Psychiatry, 54*, 1031–1037.

Filipek, P.A., Accardo, P.J., Ashwal, S., Baranek, G.T., Cook, E.H., Dawson, G., et al. (2000). Practice parameters: Screening and diagnosis of autism. Report of the Quality Standards Subcommittee of the American Academy of Neurology and the Child Neurology Society. *Neurology, 55*, 468–479.

Gillott, A., Furniss, F., Walter, A. (2001). Anxiety in high-functioning children with autism. *Autism, 5*, 277–286.

Gordon, C.T., Rapoport, J.L., Hamburger, S.D., State, R.C., Mannheim, G.B. (1992). Differential response of seven subjects with autistic disorder to clomipramine and desipramine. *American Journal of Psychiatry, 149*, 363–366.

Gordon, C.T., State, R.C., Nelson, J.E., Hamburger, S.D., Rapoport, J.L. (1993). A double-blind comparison of clomipramine, desipramine, and placebo in the treatment of autistic disorder. *Archives of General Psychiatry, 50*, 441–447.

Grados, M., Scahill, L., Riddle, M.A. (1999). Pharmacotherapy in children and adolescents with obsessive-compulsive disorder. *Child and Adolescent Psychiatric Clinics of North America, 8*, 617–634.

Greenspan, S.I., Wieder, S. (1997). Developmental patterns and outcomes in infants and children with disorders in relating and communicating: a chart review of 200 cases of children with autistic spectrum diagnoses. *The Journal of Developmental and Learning Disorders, 1*, 87–141.

Handen, B.L., Feldman, H.M., Lurier, A., Murray, P.J.H. (1999). Efficacy of methylphenidate among preschool children with developmental disabilities and ADHD. *Journal of the American Academy of Child and Adolescent Psychiatry, 38*(7), 805–812.

Harris, S.L., Powers, M.D. (1984). Behavior therapists look at the impact of an autistic child on the family system. In Schopler, E., Mesibov, G.B. (Eds.), *The Effects of Autism on the Family* (pp. 207–224). New York, NY: Plenum Press.

Harris, S.L., Handelman, J.S., Arnold, M.S., Gordon, R.F. (2000). The Douglass Developmental Disabilities Center: Two models of service delivery. In Handelman, J.S., Harris, S.L. (Eds.), *Preschool Education Programs for Children with Autism* (2nd ed.) (pp. 233–260). Austin, TX: Pro-Ed.

Hibbs, E.D., Jensen, P.S. (Eds.) (1996). *Psychosocial Treatments for Child and Adolescent Disorders: Empirically Based Strategies for Clinical Practice.* Washington, D.C. : American Psychological Association.

Hurth, J., Shaw, E., Izeman, S.G., Whaley, K., Rogers, S.J. (1999). Areas of agreement about effective practices among programs serving young children with autism spectrum disorders. *Infants and Young Children, 12*(2), 17–26.

Ingersoll, B., Stahmer, A.C., Schreibman, L. (2001). Differential treatment outcomes for children with autistic spectrum disorder based on level of peer social avoidance. *Journal of Autism and Developmental Disorders.*

Kamps, D.M., Leonard, B.R., Vernon, S., Dugan, E.P., Delquadri, J. (1992). Teaching social skills to students with autism to increase peer interactions in an integrated first-grade classroom. *Journal of Applied Behavior Analysis, 25*, 281–288.

Kamps, D.M., Barbetta, P.M., Leonard, B.R., Delquadri, J. (1994). Classwork peer tutoring: An integration strategy to improve reading skills and promote peer interactions among students with autism and general education peers. *Journal of Applied Behavior Analysis, 27*, 49–61.

Keller, M.B., Ryan, N.D., Strober, M., Klein, R.G., Kutcher, S.P., Birmaher, B., et al. (2001). Efficacy of paroxetine in the treatment of adolescent major depression: a randomized, controlled trial. *Journal of the American Academy of Child and Adolescent Psychiatry, 40,* 762–772.

Kim, J.A., Szatmari, P., Bryson, S.E., et al. (2000). The prevalence of anxiety and mood problems among children with autism and Asperger syndrome. *Autism, 4,* 117–132.

Klin, A., Sparrow, S.S., Volkmar, F.R., Cicchetti, D.V., Rourke, B.P. (1995). Asperger syndrome. In Rourke, B.P. (Ed.), *Syndrome of Nonverbal Learning Disabilities: Neurodevelopmental Manifestations (pp. 93–118).* New York, NY: Guilford Press.

Klin, A., Sparrow, S.S., Marans, W.D., Carter, A., Volkmar, F.R. (2000). Assessment issues in children and adolescents with Asperger Syndrome. In Klin, A., Volkmar, F.R., Sparrow, S.S. (Eds.), *Asperger Syndrome* (pp. 309–339). New York, NY: The Guilford Press.

Klin, A., Volkmar, F.R. (2000). Treatment and intervention guidelines for individuals with Asperger Syndrome. In Klin, A., Volkmar, F.R., Sparrow, S.S. (Eds.), *Asperger Syndrome* (pp. 340–366). New York, NY: The Guilford Press.

Klin, A., Volkmar, F.R., Sparrow, S.S. (Eds.) (2000). *Asperger Syndrome.* New York, NY: The Guilford Press.

Koegel, R.L., Frea, W.D. (1993). Treatment of social behavior in autism through the modification of pivotal social skills. *Journal of Applied Behavior Analysis, 26,* 369–377.

Koegel, L.K., Koegel, R.L., Kellegrew, D., Mullen, K. (1996). Parent education for prevention and reduction of severe problem behaviors. In Koegel, L.K., Koegel, R.L., Dunlap, G. (Eds.), *Positive Behavioral Support: Including People with Difficult Behavior in the Community* (pp. 3–30). Baltimore, MD: Brookes Publishing.

Koegel, L.K., Koegel, R.L., Harrower, J.K., Carter, C.M. (1999). Pivotal response intervention I: Overview of approach. *Journal of the Association for the Severely Handicapped, 24,* 174–185.

Lonigan, C.J., Elbert, J.C., Johnson, S.B. (1998). Empirically supported psychosocial interventions for children: An overview. *Journal of Clinical Child Psychology, 27,* 138–145.

Lovaas, O.I. (1987). Behavioral treatment and normal educational and intellectual functioning in young autistic children. *Journal of Consulting and Clinical Psychology, 55,* 3–9.

Maag, J.W., Reid, R. (1994). Attention-Deficit Hyperactivity Disorder: A Functional Approach to Assessment and Treatment. *Behavior Disorders, 201*(1), 5–23.

March, J.S., Biederman, J., Wolkow, R., Safferman, A., Mardekian, J., Cook, E.H., et al. (1998). Sertraline in children and adolescents with obsessive-compulsive disorder – a multicenter randomized controlled trial. *Journal of the American Medical Association, 280,* 1752–1756.

Marcus, L.E., Kunce, L.J., Schopler, E. (1997). Working with families. In Cohen, D.J., Bolkmar, F.R. (Eds.), *Handbook of Autism and Pervasive Developmental Disorders* (2nd Edition) (pp. 631–649). New York, NY: John Wiley & Sons.

Marcus, L.E., Schopler, E., Lord, C. (2000). TEACCH services for preschool children. In Handelman, J.S., Harris, S.L. (Eds.), *Preschool Education Programs for Children with Autism (2nd ed.).* Austin, TX: Pro-Ed.

Martin, A., Scahill, L., Klin, A., Volkmar, F. (1999). Higher-functioning pervasive developmental disorders: Rates and patterns of psychotropic drug use. *Journal of the American Academy of Child and Adolescent Psychiatry, 38,* 923–931.

Martin, A., Patzer, D.K., Volkmar, F.R. (2000). Psychopharmacological treatment of higher-functioning Pervasive Developmental Disorders. In Klin, A., Volkmar, F.R., Sparrow, S.S. (Eds.), *Asperger Syndrome* (pp. 210–228). New York, NY: The Guilford Press.

McDougle, C.J. (1997). Psychopharmacology. In Cohen, D.J. & Volkmar, F.R. (Eds.), *Handbook of Autism and Pervasive Developmental Disorders* (pp. 707–729). New York, NY: John Wiley & Sons.

McDougle, C.J., Naylor, S.T., Cohen, D.J., Volkmar, F.R., Heninger, G.R., Price, L.H. (1996). A double-blind, placebo-controlled study of fluvoxamine in adults with autistic disorder. *Archives of General Psychiatry*, 1001–1008.

McEachin, J.J., Smith, T., Lovaas, O.I. (1993). Long-term outcome for children with autism who received early intensive behavioral treatment. *American Journal of Mental Retardation, 4*, 359–372.

McGee, G.G., Morrier, M.J., Daly, T. (2000). The Walden preschool. In Handelman, J.S., Harris, S.L. (Eds.), *Preschool Education Programs for Children with Autism (2nd ed.) (pp. 157–190)*. Austin, TX: Pro-Ed.

Mesibov, G.B., Shea, V., Adams, L.W. (2001). *Understanding Asperger Syndrome and High Functioning Autism*. New York, NY: Kluwer Academic/Plenum Publishers.

Miklowitz, D.J., Simoneau, T.L., George, E.L., Richards, J.A., Kalbag, A., Sacs-Ericsson, N., Suddath, R. (2000). Family-focused treatment of bipolar disorder: 1-year effects of a psychoeducational program in conjunction with pharmacotherapy. *Biological Psychiatry, 48*, 582–592.

Muris P., Steerneman, P., Merckelbach H., Holdrinet, I., Meesters, C. (1998). Comorbid anxiety symptoms in children with pervasive developmental disorders. *Journal of Anxiety Disorders, 12*(4), 387–393.

Myles, B. (in press). Social Skills Instruction for Children with AS. In R. DuCharme & T.P. Gullotta (Eds.). Asperger Syndrome: A Handbook for Professionals and Families. NY: Kluwer Academic/Plenum Publishers.

National Research Council (2001). *Educating Children with Autism*. Committee on Educational Interventions for Children with Autism. Division of Behavioral and Social Sciences and Education. Washington, D.C.: National Academy Press.

Ozonoff, S., Miller, J.N. (1995). Teaching theory of mind: A new approach to social skills training for individuals with autism. *Journal of Autism and Developmental Disorders, 25*, 415–433.

Ozonoff, S., Cathcart, K. (1998). Effectiveness of a home program intervention for young children with autism. Journal of Autism and Developmental Disorders, 28(1), 25–35.

Penn, D.L., Mueser, K.T. (1996). Research update on the psychosocial treatment of schizophrenia. *American Journal of Psychiatry, 153*, 607–617.

Pfeiffer, S.I., Norton, J., Nelson, L., Schott, S. (1995). Efficacy of vitamin-B6 and magnesium in the treatment of autism—A methodology review and summary of outcomes. *Journal of Autism and Developmental Disorders, 25*, 481–493.

Posey, D.J., McDougle, C.J. (2000). The pharmacotherapy of target symptoms associated with Autistic Disorder and other Pervasive Developmental Disorders. *Harvard Review Psychiatry, 8*, 45–63.

Quintana, H., Birmaher, B., Stedge, D., Lennon, S., Freed, J., Bridge, J. (1995). Use of methylphenidate in the treatment of children with autistic disorder. *Journal of Autism and Developmental Disorders, 25*, 2830294.

Research Units on Pediatric Psychopharmacology (RUPP) Autism Network (2002). Risperidone in children with autism and serious behavioral problems. *The New England Journal of Medicine, 347*, 314–321.

Research Units on Pediatric Psychopharmacology (RUPP) Anxiety Study Group (2001). Fluvoxamine for the treatment of anxiety disorders in children and adolescents. *The New England Journal of Medicine, 17*, 1279–1285.

Riddle, M.A., Bernstein, G.A., Cook, E.H., Leonard, H.L., March, J.S., Swanson, J.M. (1999). Anxiolytics, adrenergic agents, and naltrexone. *Journal of the American Academy of Child and Adolescent Psychiatry, 38*(5), 546–556.

Riddle, M.A., Scahill, L., King, R.A., Hardin, M.T., Anderson, G.M., Ort, S.I., et al. (1992). Double-blind, crossover trial of fluoxetine and placebo in children and adolescents with obsessive-compulsive disorder. *Journal of the American Academy of Child and Adolescent Psychiatry, 31*, 1062–1069.

Rogers, S.J. (1998). Empirically supported treatments for young children with autism. *Journal of Clinical Child Psychology, 27*, 168–179.

Rogers, S.J. (2000). Interventions that facilitate socialization in children with autism. *Journal of Autism and Developmental Disorders, 30*(5), 399–409.

Rogers, S.J., Hall, T., Osaki, D., Reaven, J., Herbison, J. (2000). The Denver model: A comprehensive, integrated educational approach to young children with autism and their families. In Handelman, J.S., Harris, S.L. (Eds.), *Preschool Education Programs for Children with Autism (2nd ed.)*, (pp. 95–133). Austin, TX: Pro-Ed.

Sanchez, L.D., Campbell, M., Small, A.M., Cueva, J.E., Armenteros, J.L., Adams, P.B. (1996). A pilot study of clomipramine in young autistic children. *Journal of the American Academy of Child and Adolescent Psychiatry, 35*, 537–544.

Scahill, L., Chappell, P.B., Kim, Y.S., Schultz, R.T., Katsovich, L., Shepherd, E., et al. (2001). A placebo-controlled study of guanfacine in the treatment of children with tic disorders and attention deficit hyperactivity disorder. *American Journal of Psychiatry, 158*(7), 1067–1074.

Scahill, L., Riddle, M.A., King, R.A., Hardin, M.T., Rasmusson, A, Makuch, R.W., et al. (1997). Fluoxetine has no marked effect on tic symptoms in patients with Tourette syndrome: a double-blind, placebo-controlled study. *Journal of Child and Adolescent Psychopharmacology, 7*, 75–85.

Schreibman, L. (1997). Theoretical perspectives on behavioral intervention for individual with autism. In Cohen, D.J., Bolkmar, F.R. (Eds.), *Handbook of Autism and Pervasive Developmental Disorders (2nd Edition)* (pp. 920–933). New York, NY: John Wiley & Sons.

Sheinkopf, S.J., Siegel, B. (1998). Home-based behavioral treatment of young children with autism. *Journal of Autism and Developmental Disabilities, 28*, 15–23.

Siegel, B. (1996). *The World of the Autistic Child: Understanding and Treating Autistic Spectrum Disorders.* New York, NY: Oxford University Press.

Smith, T. (1999). Outcome of early intervention for children with autism. *Clinical Psychology: Science and Practice, 6*, 33–49.

Smith, T., Groen, A.D., Wynn, J.W. (2000). A randomized trial of intensive early intervention for children with pervasive developmental disorder. *American Journal on Mental Retardation, 5*(4), 269–285.

Sofronoff, K., Farbotko, M. (2002). The effectiveness of parent management training to increase self-efficacy in parents of children with Asperger syndrome. *Autism, 6*(3), 271–286.

Strain, P.S., Cordisco, L. (1994). LEAP preschool. In Handelman, J.S., Harris, S.L. (Eds.), *Preschool Education Programs for Children with Autism (2nd ed.)*, (pp. 225–244). Austin, TX: Pro-Ed.

Unis, A.S., Munson, J.A., Rogers, S.J., Goldson, E., Osterling, J., Gabriels, R., Abbott, R.D., Dawson, G. (2002). A randomized, double-blind, placebo-controlled trial of porcine versus synthetic secretin for reducing symptoms of autism. *Journal of the American Academy of Child and Adolescent Psychiatry, 41*(11), 1315–1321.

Wagner, K.D. (2001). Generalized anxiety disorder in children and adolescents. *Psychiatry Clinics of North America, 24*, 139–153.

Wilens, T.E. (2001). Pharmacologic management of Attention-Deficit/Hyperactivity Disorder. *The Economics of Neuroscience, 3*(4), 54–59.

Zollweg, W., Palm, D., Vance V. (1997). The efficacy of auditory integration training: A double blind study. *American Journal of Audiology, 6*, 39–47.

Chapter 5

Identifying and Preventing the Risks for Victimization of Children with Asperger Syndrome

Liza Little

This chapter addresses the unique risk factors for victimization of children with Asperger Syndrome (AS) at the individual child, family, and community levels. Suggestions and strategies are offered for the assessment and primary prevention of victimization in this population.

Children who are both disabled and maltreated may be among the most vulnerable segments in our population (Ammerman, 1997; Sullivan & Knutson, 2000; National Center on Child Abuse and Neglect, 1993). Children with disabilities are two to three times more likely to be abused or neglected in their homes, than are non-disabled children (NCCAN, 1993; Sullivan & Knutson, 1998; 2000). Among children with disabilities, children with Autism–spectrum disorders are at particular risk (Sullivan & Knutson, 2000).

Children with Autism-spectrum disorders such as AS are an understudied population. Due to better diagnosis there are increasing numbers of children receiving the diagnosis that many consider to be a mild form of or a variant of autism. Children with AS have problems with reciprocal social interaction and communication, and stereotyped, repetitive interests and behaviors. Therefore, children with AS have limited ability to take part in reciprocal communication and have difficulties understanding the rules of communication reflected in deficits in language pragmatics (Lainhart, 1999). Although the child with AS may be very verbal, he/she may also have significant trouble with basic problem solving and critical thinking. Due to problems with sensory integration, children with AS may also have difficulties with emotional reactivity, and modulation (Barnhill, 2001).

Children with AS may suffer "intersecting oppressions" (Richie, 1997); they are easy targets because of the seriousness of their social skills deficits, the invisibility of their difficulties (they look like normal children), and the lack of public and professional understanding of the syndrome. Failure by professionals to recognize that some children are more vulnerable to victimization than others may discourage the availability, and adaptability of interventions that focus on prevention and treatment.

Prevalence of Victimization

Children with autism disorders have a relative risk for victimization by caregivers that is one of the highest among children with disabilities (Sullivan & Knutson, 1998; 2000). In one of the largest, well controlled, epidemiological studies of maltreated children with disabilities, children with behavioral disorders and children with autism disorders were seven times more likely to be physically and emotionally abused, and neglected in their homes, and five times more likely to be sexually abused than were children with communication, orthopedic, intellectual or learning disabilities, suggesting a possible high relative risk for children with AS (Sullivan & Knutson, 2000).

In a recent study of maternal discipline of children with AS, rates of maternal verbal aggression (screaming and yelling, swearing, threatening to kick the child out, and calling the child names), were found to be higher than those reported by parents in a gallop poll survey of children in the general population (Little, 2002a). At the same time, rates of physical methods of discipline such as slapping, pinching and shaking the child, were also elevated (Little, 2002a). In this study of 411 mothers of children with AS, mothers of ten year olds reported using verbal or psychological aggression the most (33 times a year), and mothers of four year olds with AS reported using spanking on the bottom with a hand or slapping the most (14 times in the last year). As children with AS got older, almost all forms of discipline declined. Notable exceptions were threatening to send the child away, which peaked in the teen years, calling the child dumb or lazy, which peeked in preteen years and remained elevated, and finally, hitting the child with a hard object such as a belt, although a very rare occurrence, was as common for younger children as it was for older children (Little, 2002a).

Victimization of the child with AS can also occur by peers and siblings, inside or outside of the home. Mothers of children with AS have reported significant rates of peer and sibling bullying and assault, gang attacks, and social exclusion by peers (Little, 2002b). Peer and sibling assault rates were eight times higher for the children with AS than for a large sample of youth in an internet safety study (Finkelhor, Mitchell, & Walak, 2000). Gang attacks, or attacks by groups of children, although very rare in the general population, were five times higher for children with AS (Little, 2002b).

Professionals may not routinely include social exclusion by peers, as a significant form of victimization when they screen children, but for children with AS, it is an important form of victimization. Mothers of children with AS reported that 33% of their children with AS had not been to a birthday party in the last year, a third were reported to be sitting alone every day at lunch, and more than half were almost always picked last for teams by their peers (Little, 2002b). Although these findings are preliminary, they suggest that children with AS may be at significant risk for multiple types of victimization.

There is little empirical research on the maltreatment of children with AS, even though their numbers are rising and they are receiving growing national attention (Rapin, 2002). To what extent children and youth with AS may be victims of other crimes such as street or internet crimes, or accused of committing crimes that they were unaware of is unknown. Further research in these areas is necessary.

One of the reasons for the lack of information regarding the prevalence of victimization is because basic child welfare investigative procedures of maltreated children often fail to document whether a child has a disability, and some states do not even recognize AS as a disability, therefore children with less well known disabilities, such as AS, are even less likely to be identified. Only 19 states in the U.S. currently require records on disability status when a complaint of child maltreatment is made (NCCAN, 2001). Children with disabilities are over-represented in the child welfare system, but the extent of the over representation is not known (Bruhn, 2002). The inability of professionals to recognize the special risk of certain children may compromise the efficacy of interventions when they are available (Gazelle & Ladd, 2002; Mansell, Sobsey, & Moskal, 1998).

Assessing Risk Factors for Children with Asperger Syndrome

Victimization of a child with AS can take place anywhere from the home to the school bus, to the internet, be perpetrated by a variety of offenders, and involve a number of different types of victimization. Victimization can occur by known adults and strangers, figures of authority, and peers and siblings. Peer and sibling victimization can include physical as well as relational victimization where threats, ridicule, and manipulations occur (Crick, Casas, & Nelson, 2002). Victimization can occur at any developmental age or stage.

The child with AS may experience multiple forms of victimization. He/she may be bullied or ridiculed at school, shunned on the bus ride home, yelled at or slapped by a caregiver at home, and be coping with multiple stressors that extend from interactions in his/her family, to school peers, teachers, and the greater community. Parents of some children with AS may be struggling as well, confronting the barriers to obtaining services for their child, struggling to understand how to provide adequate care, get respite breaks, and manage families, marriages, and jobs. Parents may feel victimized. Teachers and school systems can feel oppressed by resource limitations, inclusionary regulations, and lack of training (Weinberg, 1997). The pressure for schools to create services for children with less-well-known disabilities while being provided with limited resources cannot be underestimated.

Victimization of children with AS is best assessed by examining the possibility for multiple determinants occurring at the different levels of the systems influencing the child. These include the individual child, the child's family, and the child's community (Belsky, 1993). These factors create the context for child maltreatment and victimization and are often intertwined (Belsky, 1993; Grauerholz, 2000). Assessing for multiple determinants is also critical in the consideration of maltreatment because it helps to frame treatment and prevention in terms of multiple perspectives, and is more likely to generate a more systemic view, minimize over interpretation , and prevent the focus on single causes or the exclusive focus on the individual child with AS (Llewellyn & Hogan, 2000; Sullivan & Cork, 1998). Taking multiple perspectives also helps to generate compassion and minimize blame.

Individual Risk Factors for Children with Asperger Syndrome

Children with AS usually have some degree of qualitative impairments in social interaction secondary to impaired use of nonverbal behaviors to regulate interpersonal communication, difficulties developing age appropriate peer relations, lack of spontaneous interest in sharing experience with others, and a lack of emotional reciprocity (Klin, Volkmar & Sparrow, 2000). This may lead to an inability or lack of desire to interact with peers, poor interpretation of social cues and socially and emotionally inappropriate responses. In addition, children with AS may also have restricted, repetitive patterns of behavior, interests and activities, and be inflexible to changes in their routines. These limitations create problems with sharing joint activities with peers, basic play, or taking a trip with the family.

The child with AS may also have speech and language difficulties such as odd prosody, unusual voice characteristics, and impaired comprehension of the literal and implied meanings of things. They may gesture infrequently, be physically clumsy, have a limited number of facial expressions, and have problems with physical proximity including bumping into others (Bauer, 1999). Children with AS tend to be socially isolated and can be socially intrusive at times. They have difficulty changing their behavior to fit the needs of their environment.

These very characteristics of AS increase the child's *target vulnerability*, *target gratifiability*, and *target antagonism* to offenders (Finkelhor & Asdigian, 1996, p. 6). Target *vulnerability* refers to characteristics of victims that increase their risk because they compromise the person's ability to resist or deter victimization and thus make them easier targets for offenders (Finkelhor & Asdigian, 1996). A typical example would be small physical stature or physical weakness. For the child with AS, The inability to decipher social cues, read facial expressions, or pick up a certain tone of voice would also be examples of target vulnerabilities. The child with AS may have difficulty recognizing the verbal and nonverbal behaviors of a bully, or saying no to a request. In social situations the youth with AS is more likely to be unaware of many of the cues that alert others to the possibility of criminal victimization or that a situation is unsafe. These vulnerabilities make it more difficult for the child with AS to deter a bully, assuage an abusive parent, or seek help.

On the other hand, the sweet, naive, friendly, innocence, and literalness, that many children with AS exhibit may make them more appealing targets to offenders. These are qualities or attributes that an offender may find gratifying and exploit. The child with AS who is asked to do something inappropriate in exchange for a promise of friendship, for example, is an example of *target gratifiability*. The child with AS is picked because the offender knows s/he can manipulate the child's gullibility (Finkelhor & Asdigian, 1996).

Target antagonism refers to the attributes a child may have that actually antagonize or arouse anger in an offender (Finkelhor & Asdigian, 1996). In the case of parental harsh discipline or assault, the child's disability-specific behaviors, or disobedience, may be perceived as antagonizing, or as a burden and provoke abuse. Aggressive behavior and withdrawal (not uncommon to children with AS) can be construed as antagonistic and lead to rejection and victimization. The child with AS may have specific rituals and routines he/she insists on following that are perceived as oppositional by peers and adults alike. The intensity of the child's inflexibility and emotional reactivity can tax the most compassionate parent or professional (Greene, 1998).

Target vulnerability, gratifiability, and antagonism, don't disappear with age. Individual risk factors shift with developmental age and can become even more pronounced with years. The characteristics of AS become more pronounced as the demands for more sophisticated and complex social skills increase. A lack of friends in elementary school may be less noticeable than a lack of friends in high school. For the adolescent with AS, victimization may not stop. In fact, parents have reported greater social exclusion for adolescents with AS by their peers (Little, 2000b). Relationally victimizing behaviors become more sophisticated in adolescence when children can begin to use tactics such as spreading rumors, stealing boyfriends, or telling secrets to others (Crick, Casas, & Nelson, 2002). The clinical reports that point to higher rates of depression for adolescents with AS suggest that this may be due to the greater awareness of the adolescent with AS of his/her differences and limitations (Barnhill, 2001; Ghaziuddin, Weidmer, & Ghaziuddin, 1998).

Family Risk Factors

Children with AS whose families have multiple stressors are at greater potential risk for abuse and neglect. Factors such as poverty, a parent with mental or physical illness, domestic violence, drug and alcohol abuse, single parent status, or unemployment, are all associated with a greater risk for child maltreatment (Committee on Child Abuse & Neglect, 2001; Streeck-Fischer, & van der Kolk, 2000; Sullivan & Knutson, 2000). Findings suggest that rates of depression, and help seeking for mothers of children with neurocognitive disorders such as attention deficit hyperactivity disorder, and AS are significant (Lewis-Abney, 1993; Little, 2002c; McCormick, 1995, Mick, Santangelo, Wypij, & Biederman, 2000). In a recent study of 103 couples who had children with AS, mothers were significantly more likely to be taking medication for depression and seeking professional help for themselves than their spouses. Mothers were also more likely to report feeling more pessimistic about their child's future and to report more personal and family stress in relationship to their child than their spouses (Little, 2002c). High parental stress may in fact, increase the likelihood for abuse.

Family factors such as ineffective parenting skills and the use of harsh discipline may also put a child with AS at risk for maltreatment (DePanfilis, 1998; Little, 2002a; Straus, 2000). The literature on the use of spanking, corporal punishment, and even verbal aggression and threats suggests that these methods only work in the short run to produce compliance, and have many negative health outcomes for the child when used persistently (Straus & Stewart, 1999; Straus, 2000). Recent research indicates that harsh parental discipline and child abuse is associated with the development of conduct disorders in children (Sullivan & Knutson, 1998). Children with AS may be labeled as having a conduct disorder because of their behavioral issues, but it is important to sort out if the conduct disorder is provoked by appropriate caregiver discipline or issues inherent to the expression of the disability. The question of whether it is the child's disability that provokes the maltreatment, the maltreatment that creates the secondary pathology such as the conduct problems, are critical questions for clinicians when assessing any child with a disability, and particularly those with behavioral control issues (Mitchell & Buchele-Ash, 2000). Understanding that the relationship between AS, and victimization is not unidirectional can help to decrease stereotyping and bias about children with AS.

Clinical reports suggest that parents of children with AS do have concerns with basic parenting skills from addressing behavior control (Greene, 1998), to how to teach day-to-day social skills. Assessing the parenting skills of a parent of a child with AS takes on a different meaning because many of the social skills that children with AS are lacking, are not easy to teach by the most well meaning adult or professional.

The child maltreatment literature indicates that another major risk factor for youth victimization in the family is the lack of guardianship or supervision by caregivers of children in their homes and communities (Finkelhor & Asdigian, 1996). Child neglect, one of the most common forms of child maltreatment for children with disabilities, often involves issues related to inadequate child supervision.

Guardianship issues can occur at the family or community level. When children spend a lot of time alone or apart from the family or other caring figures, it reduces the possibility of parental supervision or "guardianship" that would protect the child from possible victimization (Finkelhor & Asdigian, 1996). Findings from child abuse studies indicate that lack of adult supervision can be a risk factor for child sexual abuse; and family isolation, a risk factor for child physical abuse (Finkelhor & Asdigian, 1996). Lack of child supervision can also extend to more seemingly benign but possibly dangerous situations such as lack of internet supervision (Finkelhor, Mitchell & Walak, 2000). Recent findings suggest that many children are sexually solicited over the internet and in a growing number of cases this has led to dangerous consequences for the child (Finkelhor, Mitchell & Walak, 2000). Lack of supervision can also extend during the school day, at recess, on the bus, and after school, or in periods when children have free time. These are often prime times for victimization by peers to occur (Hazler, Miller, Carny & Green, 2001).

Children with AS require careful supervision and often prefer to be alone. They enjoy spending time engaging in interests that are often solitary, or spend time alone to decrease the sensory overload in their environments, and manage their social anxiety. Parents of children with AS may need to be careful not to leave their child alone, too often. Many children and young adults with AS are also attracted to the internet as a significant means to establishing contacts and friendships outside their families. Virtual relationships are often easier for individuals who have difficulty with understanding nonverbal behavior and communication. In fact, the stereotype of the child with AS being a computer or electronics "nerd" is not uncommon. Children who spend a lot of time on the internet, are at greater risk for sexual solicitation and are unlikely to tell their parents (Finkelhor, Mitchell & Walak, 2000). For these reasons it is important for clinicians and professionals to educate parents and screen for possible internet exposure when working with a child with AS.

Another type of guardianship issue specific to children with AS is the ease with which children with AS get lost and have difficulties negotiating their physical environments (Rourke, 1995). The less familiar the environment, the greater the risk for getting lost will be. Parents and professionals may make assumptions about safety that are not warranted for the child with AS, even at developmental stages where getting lost would not ordinarily be an issue.

Community Risk Factors

There are a number of systems contributions to the increased risk for maltreatment of children with AS. One of the most important is the lack of understanding and awareness of well-meaning adults and professionals. Attitudes held by the community towards individuals that are different are also potential contributors to victimization risk. Early research in the field of disabilities and social psychology demonstrated that people tend to tolerate certain types of disabilities better than others. People tend to treat individuals who are blind and deaf better, than those with mental illness, for instance. People who are the least likely to be treated tolerantly are those individuals who think, talk, or act differently (Tringo, 1970). This suggests that society as a whole, is less tolerant and this intolerance can sow the seeds of victimization for individuals with social skills deficits and behavioral problems such as individuals with AS.

Recent research shows that teachers' perceptions of the severity of a child's disability influence their attitudes toward students with disabilities in their classrooms. Children with hidden disabilities, including learning disabilities (such as AS), are more likely to engender intolerance in teachers than children with more obvious disabilities, such as orthopedic disabilities, or Downs Syndrome (Cook, 2001). The implication here is that children and youth with AS may be less accepted because they sometimes act and communicate differently and that there are social prejudices that even professionals can hold.

Medical and mental health systems can increase children's vulnerability to maltreatment by not providing adequate care to meet the unique needs of a child with AS (Mitchell & Buchele-Ash, 2000). For example, going over a standard adolescent questionnaire on health habits, which is fairly routine for many pediatric practices, requires understanding AS in order to make the questionnaire a useful, valid and reliable experience. Children with AS are very literal, and if the question reads "have you ever run away from home" they may answer "yes" because they "ran in the direction away from their home, once". If the questionnaire asks, "do you have bleeding problems" the child with AS may respond positively because it's always a problem when he/she gets a cut. This means that medical professionals need to use secondary sources such as parents and teachers to confirm the responses and experiences of the adolescent with As as well as educating themselves about the syndrome.

The diagnosis of AS may go unrecognized in mental health settings, especially if other mental health diagnoses co-exist (Burger & Lang, 1998; Gillberg & Billstedt, 2000; Raja & Azzoni, 2000). Misdiagnoses can lead to unintended iatrogenic harm to the individual with AS and their families. Some of the odd and unusual features of individuals with AS may be mistaken for schizophrenia, for instance, and several clinical features of AS may be confused with signs of depression. At baseline many individuals with AS who are not depressed are quiet, socially withdrawn, and have flattish facial expressions (Lainhart, 1999).

Educational systems can inadvertently increase the risk for victimization of children with AS if they don't provide education that is adequate for preparing the child with AS for their day-to-day life. Individualizing the education plans for children with AS that take into account their unique challenges, would help to prevent the occurrence of a "one shoe fits all" approach to special education or placing them in settings with children with major emotional disorders that may be counterproductive to the child with AS (Klin, Volkmar, & Sparrow, 2000). The availability of resources for children with AS such as adequate social skills training, pragmatics, and individualized, educational supports, is another important issue in the prevention of victimization of children with AS. Resources may be lacking in schools overwhelmed with children with more common special needs (Little, 2002d).

School systems are increasingly being confronted with the problem of school violence, peer bullying, and coercive power dynamics in which a bully, which can be a child, teacher, or other staff member of the school abusively coerces others repeatedly through humiliation and mockery (Twemlow, Fonagy, & Sacco, 2001). One response to these problems has been the adoption of zero-tolerance policies to prevent school violence. These policies however, do not address the special issues of children who have AS (Huchet, 2001). Inflexible enforcement could be considered abusive treatment of the child with AS. Children with AS are particularly vulnerable to zero tolerance policies in their schools because of the seriousness of their social skills and executive function deficits. A child with AS may break a rule and have no idea what he/she has done wrong or why they are punished for it. The child with AS may be set up by another child, to commit an infraction without the child with AS understanding their role. The following situation reported by a parent provides an example: An eighth grade girl with AS is told by a male peer, that he will be her boyfriend if she downloads some "pictures" for him from the school computer. The girl complies, eager to have a friend. The pictures turn out to be pornographic, the girl naively shows the pictures to her parents and tells them the story, and the parents then report it to the school. The girl is then suspended and her school computer privileges are withdrawn for the rest of the school year. The girl is devastated by the punishment because she had no idea that what she was doing was wrong. Her peers ridicule her for her "naiveté." Her parent's feel victimized because the school does not take into account the child's AS.

Other community factors that may contribute to increasing the risk for victimization for children with AS may occur when social service systems that provide services to children with disabilities are separate from child protective systems, and differ in their eligibility requirements and age cut off. This situation places the child with AS at risk for "falling through the cracks" and not receiving the care he/she needs. Therefore the case protection model may be inadequate to meet this child's needs (Klin, Volkmar & Sparrow, 2000).

Impact of Victimization

Children with AS who have been exposed to chronic childhood trauma will have more difficulties with the capacity for a normal developmental trajectory and may experience a host of devastating symptoms. The impact of abuse on children with neurodevelopmental disabilities is just as devastating as it is for children without disabilities (Shirk & Eltz, 1998). The development of anxious attachments, posttraumatic stress disorder, anxiety and depression are common. Problems with oppositional behavior, emotional self-regulation, and regulation of affect, impulse control, and aggression towards self and others may also develop (Streek-Fischer & van der Kolk, 2000; Mullen, Martin, Anderson, Romans, & Herbison, 1996).

Children with AS have difficulty communicating and understanding their experiences, thus clinicians have to be especially vigilant to assess the development of any self-harming behaviors in the child or adolescent with AS. Unfortunately, in the past these behaviors have been commonly attributed to the disability status of a child, and rarely viewed as a symptom of possible abuse as they are in children without disabilities (Downie, 2001; Mansell et al., 1998).

Some abuse issues may be compounded for the child with AS by factors related to the disability. The experience of social isolation, dependency on others, particularly family members, can increase the child's anxiety, anger, and fear of retaliation and abandonment (Mansell et al., 1998). Inadequate knowledge and comfort with sexuality and normative social behavior accompanied by changes in hormones, and the ability to understand what are safe and unsafe environments, may complicate the adolescent with AS's understanding of his/her abuse (Clees & Gast, 1994; Mansell et al., 1998). Trauma magnifies communication problems in individuals with neuro-developmental disabilities. These children may be more confused and have a greater difficulty understanding their abuse and communicating about it (Mansell et al., 1998). One might surmise, therefore, that the child with AS who has difficulties identifying feelings, and understanding nonverbal behavior, will have significant difficulties communicating about abuse that has occurred. There may be a higher likelihood of repressing and burying traumatic events since feelings tend to overwhelm them in every day coping with life events.

Preventing the Victimization of Children with Asperger Syndrome

There is a small literature on treatment programs for preventing the victimization of individuals with disabilities, little on the empirical evidence for efficacy outcomes, and virtually no information on the treatment of traumatized children with AS (Clees & Gast, 1994; Mazzucchelli, 2001; Moturella, 1998; Orelove et al., 1999). This is disappointing as the effective treatment for any child with a disability, such as AS should be derived from empirical outcomes. The few programs that are described tend to address strangers, abductions, and sexual abuse, and many are designed for adults with developmental disabilities (Mazzucchelli, 2001). There is a sizeable gap between clinical practice and empirical outcome studies that demonstrate their effectiveness with children with disabilities. This gap also extends to determining the efficacy for parent education programs for caregivers who abuse their children (Reppucci, Britner, & Woolard, 1997; Shirk & Eltz, 1998).

Children with disabilities who have been maltreated also face gaps in services, unavailable or inaccessible therapy, and counseling, and services that are not modified for the individual child (Mansell et al., 1998). Children with AS are no exception and parents of children with AS report concerns about the victimization of their children, the lack of availability of resources, and the relative "unhelpfulness" of existing mental health resources (Little, 2002d).

Teachers, counselors, parents, nurses, doctors, and caseworkers all need to work together to prevent the victimization of children with AS. Prevention efforts need to target the different adults in various parts of the individual child's life to foster collaboration across all professions and individuals. If collaboration is to occur, adults in the life of a child with AS have to be able to recognize when victimization occurs.

Child Interventions

All clinicians working to prevent victimization of children with AS need to communicate the message that "everyone has the right to feel safe," and "nothing is so bad that we can't talk with someone about it" (Mazzucchelli, 2001, p. 115). Although it is the responsibility of adults to protect children from victimization, as children grow older, basic safety should be taught to all youth. Junior high school children and adolescents with AS need to learn how to recognize unsafe situations, the importance of taking action in unsafe situations, and how to use a network of safe individuals to get help. They need explicit practice with learning how to problem solve and develop strategies to help keep safe. The information needs to be given in a manner in which is meaningful to the youth with AS. Children with AS have difficulties understanding social interaction and may be unaware of the cues that alert others to the possibility of criminal or abusive behavior. Their desire for friendship and a learning history that is often based on getting reinforced for compliance, may make it more difficult for them to refuse an abusive request. Children with AS have difficulties generalizing, and often struggle with "black and white thinking", so how the information is presented are very important. This means that counselors, teachers, and parents need to think through common types of scenarios the child is likely to encounter and discuss them with the child. It is impossible to anticipate the huge variety of situations, so learning to use a problem solving attitude will help the child/adolescent with readiness for the unexpected.

Programs such as the Feel Safe (Mazzucchelli, 2001), and the Multidimensional Bullying Identification Model (Marini, Fairbairn & Zuber, 2001) although targeted for individuals with developmental disabilities could be used and modified for youth with AS. These programs target certain skills such as how to recognize an unsafe situation or the characteristics of a bully and common school bullying situations, the importance of taking action in unsafe situations, how to develop a network of personal confidants, self-assertion skills, and problem solving to develop strategies to keep safe (Marini, Fairbairn & Zuber, 2001; Mazzucchelli, 2001). Using curriculum material in a range of medias, using group instruction, modeling, and role plays, and providing feedback and shaping skill development by the use of praise for adaptive efforts are key strategies to goal attainment. Both the Feel Safe program, and the Multidimensional Bullying Identification Model have undergone preliminary testing for efficacy and are showing positive, measurable, outcomes (Marini, Fairbairn & Zuber, 2001; Mazzucchelli, 2001).

Programs that focus on teaching children to protect themselves are not recommended for younger children. The responsibility for protection should never be placed on the younger child and efforts should be made to address the total social ecology of the child's experience (Orelove, Hollahan, & Myles, 2000).

Although child abductions are actually very rare compared to many other forms of child victimization, older children with AS should know the common lures that stranger-predators use with abductions such as "will you help me find my lost pet," "your house is on fire, your family is having an emergency . . . I'll take you home, get in the car with me . . . " and practice basic safety strategies for street safety. Likewise, children with AS need to be taught how to use the phone, to carry identification cards with them, and be able to identify safe adults who she/he can talk with in the event of difficulty.

Children with AS get lost easily. When out on excursions, visiting, traveling, or shopping, the child should never be left alone and if possible, buddied up with another child who does not have AS to help the child with AS find his/her way and to help them learn from the other child. Buddy systems should be used in schools and on school buses as well. Children with AS involved with after school activities, church, or scouts, need those adults to also understand their limitations and strengths, and help to protect them from victimization Procedures should be developed and over-learning should be the goal for the child with AS.

As children with AS get older, they need to learn about dating, sex, and appropriate intimate behavior and this is not an easy task for an individual who does not understand nonverbal behavior, misjudges social cues, and does not readily "read" tone of voice, gesture, or facial expressions. Some clinicians are finding help from some of the latest reference books such as *Dating for Dummies* and *Etiquette for Idiots*. These basic primers can sometimes offer the step-by-step scripts necessary for children with AS to learn the complicated social world of interpersonal intimacy. Talking to adolescents explicitly, rehearsing safe and unsafe scenarios, practicing and role playing behavior, and discussing normal expectations for dating is vital.

Social skills training is considered to be a core requirement to any remediation program for children with AS (Klin, Volkmar & Sparrow, 2000). Although getting social skills training is no guarantee that a child will not be victimized, children with better social skills are less likely to be victimized by peers and adults (Finkelhor & Asdigian, 1996). Adolescence, in particular, occurs just at the point when hormones change, social skills become more complex, where the demand for them is much higher, and where relational victimization becomes more sophisticated (Crick et al., 2002). These changes increase the demand on limited resources in the child with AS's weakest area: relational resources. If schools continued to provide social skills training once the child with AS entered junior high or high school, victimization risks might be reduced . Creating situations where social skills can be practiced and feedback can occur are important for the youth with AS. High schools often do provide improvisation groups, debate clubs, and community service projects, where some of this practice can take place in these structured environments. Clinicians and parents may have to advocate for additional resources for the child with AS.

Family Interventions

Efforts for preventing victimization in the home by caregivers need to focus on parent education and the parenting skills specific to the child with AS, as well as reducing the stressors faced by parents raising children with AS (Little, 2002c).

Professionals working with parents of children with AS need to screen for and assess the disciplinary practices of the family and the school and the ways in which behavior control is managed. Traditional behavior methods don't work effectively with the child with AS (Greene, 1998) and thus parents and schools need assistance with workable methods in managing behavior issues with these children.

Children with AS often don't understand the mistakes they make and their cognitive rigidity makes it more difficult for them to adapt in new situations or see the situation from another perspective. Therefore, they actually don't see the "mistake", especially if it involves contextual behavior (Greene, 1998). Some of the victimization children with AS experience may occur because the adults in their world misunderstand the degree to which the child can't do what is expected, or doesn't understand what is expected, which then causes the child to become highly anxious and disruptive. Strategies that appear to work better for the child with AS are ones where parents learn how to match their expectations to their child's ability, and therefore anticipate where problems will arise for the child, and problem solve them ahead of time.

In addition, more realistic expectations allow parents to pick their battles and their goals more judiciously, which in turn reduces conflict. Parent training should include teaching parents how to use empathy and logical persuasion, or distraction and humor as alternatives to traditional disciplinary responses (Greene, 1998).

Parents need training from skilled professionals. The better the parent understands AS, the better he/she can mediate the child's emotional world before the child escalates, and respond to the limitations of the child without targeting their frustration directly on the child. This is, of course, also true for other adults in the child's world. Children with AS have major difficulties with flexibility and frustration tolerance; however, these limitations are often not obvious. AS is an invisible set of deficits and there is no tip-off for adults that this particular child has neurocognitive deficits (Greene, 1998). Uninformed adults and even peers may view the child's behavior as willful and intentional. Therefore it is critical that the adults in the child's life understand the nature of the disorder and its particular manifestations.

Any time professionals and parents set behavioral goals for the child with AS, their primary aim should be to reduce the demand for flexibility and frustration. The adults in the child's life need to focus on anticipating specific situations that may lead to inflexible or frustrating behaviors in order to prevent behavioral problems. Something as benign as having a substitute teacher unfamiliar with the child can lead to inadvertent and inappropriate treatment of the child due to unrealistic expectations.

Parents need help in learning that confronting a child with AS who is on the verge of a tantrum should be avoided since it increases the child's frustration and sense of inadequacy, and will overwhelm his/her already overburdened self control (Greene, 1998). Children with AS often describe reaching a point of incoherence when they are frustrated and confrontations usually aggravate the situation. Parents of children with AS are particularly vulnerable when they have to cope with their child's inflexibility in public, or in front of others. The issue of embarrassment and the pressure to resolve a situation quickly may lead to serious confrontations and communication breakdown. Parents need help from empathic professionals to learn how to problem solve these situations with the least amount of damage to the child and parent.

Parents also need education on the importance of supervising their child on the Internet regularly. They should be encouraged to use blocks on their child's computers, and monitor web site and chat room visits. Clinicians need to screen for Internet victimization and ask the child with AS on a regular basis, if he/she has been solicited, talk about and problem solve strategies for preventing this. In a recent report on child victimization over the Internet, a high proportion of the children in the study who had been sexually solicited did not tell their parents, and children that were most at risk for solicitation were those who spent the most time on the computer with little, if any parental monitoring (Finkelhor, Mitchell & Walak, 2000). For these reasons it is particularly important for parents of children with AS to supervise their child's internet use.

Ongoing skill building is vital for parents. Giving parents and other adults in the child's life resources such as books, web sites and support groups to avail them selves of, will also help to decrease parental stress and inadvertent victimization.

Community Interventions

School interventions have to begin with teachers recognizing what is peer bullying and what is not. Some recent evidence suggests that teachers and counselors find it difficult to recognize and label events that are forms of peer bullying and minimize bullying situations unless they include physical violence (Hazler, Miller, Carney & Green, 2001).

Worthy intervention goals of any prevention program will depend in part, on the type of victimization that is being targeted. Important goals of school intervention programs for peer victimization should include prohibiting acts of victimization, decreasing bystander tolerance, mitigating individual vulnerability, and augmenting the supports to vulnerable children through the cultivation of peer friendships (Gazelle & Ladd, 2002; Twemlow, Fonagy & Sacco, 2001). Identifying the bullies, victims and bully bystanders is an important first step (Twemlow, Fonagy & Sacco, 2001). Teachers, counselors, and education staff, need to understand which children are more at risk of getting picked on, and in the case of children with AS, understand the unique features of the disability in order to intervene effectively. Anti-bullying programs, and tolerance programs are being initiated in many schools and should be encouraged as should the education of the peers and adults in the life of the child with AS about AS. One element of any good anti-harassment intervention is education. The more the child's peers and teachers understand the child's difficulties, the more likely they are to accept and make allowances for the child. To achieve this requires more than information, it requires care giving from teachers and peers. Guidance counselors and other school professionals can develop friendship networks to help children learn how to connect with a child with AS which will provide buffering against victimization and loneliness (Gazelle & Ladd, 2002). School mental health professionals can help teachers to develop noncoercive discipline plans which will also help to prevent victimization of the child with AS because adult can be bullies too (Twemlow et al., 2001). Finally, proper screening for victimization is critical for the child with AS. Direct questioning about bullying and victimization, along with broader questions such as "who is the scariest kid at your school?", or "do you ever not want to go to school because you know your are gong to be picked on?" may illuminate ongoing bullying behavior (Twemlow et. al., 2001, p. 378). Critical to the success of these prevention efforts is the evaluation of their outcomes to ensure their utility.

Implications for Clinicians

It is important for clinicians to have information and training on Autism spectrum disorders, and AS in particular. As more and more children are diagnosed with AS, learning about their maltreatment vulnerabilities, methods for working with them, and resources in their communities, is vital to the adequate prevention of their victimization (Sullivan & Cork, 1998; Batshaw, 1997). Requesting or seeking out continuing education in this area is important (Orelove et al., 2000). Every state has an office of developmental disabilities that can provide names of agencies and institutions that do trainings and have information. Badly needed are specific treatment outcome studies that are longitudinal and not anecdotal.

Prevention is intricately linked to assessment and careful evaluation of the specifics of a potential abuse situation, assessing the family environment and parent-child relationship, and then examining other social units that interact with the family, including those of school, work, other caregivers, and friends, is crucial for a comprehensive evaluation (Clees & Gast, 1994). Monitoring multiple domains of functioning including behavioral adjustment, adaptive skills, academic skills, social and communicative skills, and the child social interaction with the family members and peers are all important. The heterogeneity of children with AS, the great variation in the degree of their neurological deficits and symptom expression and the impact that has on their personality development, and the uniqueness of their individual family situation, calls for a broad and comprehensive approach to assessment and ongoing evaluation (Ammerman, 1997). No two children or families are alike when it comes to problems, symptoms, or skill deficits. The evaluation of children with AS demands many of the same assessment procedures and tools that a clinician would use with a child without AS.

Treatment and prevention of the victimization of children with AS also has to include providing resources and education to parents, educators, legal and medical professionals, and social service caseworkers. The goals of treatment for children with AS who have been maltreated are to provide ways to make sense out of what happened (since they so often don't understand context) and to alleviate guilt, repair trust, overcome depression, and self-harming behaviors, to improve self esteem, and teach self-protective strategies (Hollins & Sinason, 2000; Mansell et al., 1998). In addition, stopping the abuse and seeing to it that all the individuals in the child's life are educated requires a high level of collaboration, coordination, and advocacy.

All treatment occurs in the context of a therapeutic relationship and the development of a therapeutic alliance with the child, family, and those working directly with the child are crucial. The development of a treatment alliance is a challenging task with children who have been abused at the hands of caregivers, peers, and other adults, and maltreated children with AS are no exception. It may, however, require a greater commitment from the clinician to engage the child with AS who has been maltreated. Clinicians will have to find ways to communicate and connect that fit the child with AS and his/her unique way of processing information and feelings. The use of explicit verbal strategies, which can be applied to problematic situations and explicit procedures for teaching of social problem solving, may be useful. Traditional insight therapy may not be a model that works best for children with AS (Gillberg & Billstedt, 2000, Rourke, 1995).

Clinicians have tremendous contributions to make in preventing the victimization of children with AS. Learning about the range of syndrome expression in AS, and the complexities of the disorder, increasing their awareness regarding child, family, and community, risk factors for victimization, identifying and correcting gaps in the services to children with AS, and developing and promoting service delivery models that meet the unique needs of these children are important goals.

Conclusion

The numbers of children receiving the diagnosis of AS are increasing nation-wide. These children suffer from significant deficits in social pragmatics and communication, emotional modulation, and critical thinking skills. Children with AS have difficulties with cognitive flexibility and frustration tolerance. These difficulties lead to a greater vulnerability for multiple forms of victimization because the deficits are invisible, because many professionals are unfamiliar with them, and because society in general, is less tolerant of people who act, speak, or think differently. Victimization of the child with AS therefore, can take place at the individual, family or community level.

Education is the single most important tool to prevention of child maltreatment. Prevention of victimization must begin with educating adults and caregivers from across disciplines on the unique features of AS, common types of difficulties the child may run into, and the effective prevention of those problems. Parents require training and education in parenting skills, managing behavior issues, and how to advocate for their child in various systems. Parents need support and empathy as they grapple with the sometimes-overwhelming issues related to raising a child in a culture that currently understands very little about their child's problems.

Education has to include school interventions that directly involve teaching the child social pragmatics all through the child's developmental trajectory, identifies the potential for victimization, and teaches basic safety skills in a meaningful way. Zero tolerance polices need to be examined carefully for potential hidden discrimination toward the child with AS who may not understand the difference between socially appropriate and inappropriate behavior.

In addition to education, research is required to better understand the unique vulnerabilities of children with AS, as well as on treatment and prevention that is empirically derived and evaluated for efficacy. Although the victimization of children with disabilities is a major public health problem, the research on the prevention and treatment of victimization of children with disabilities has taken a back seat. The research to date often lumps children with various types of disabilities into larger groups, promulgating the myth that children with disabilities need similar interventions. Children with AS do not respond to some of the more traditional forms of behavioral intervention (Greene, 1998) that have been used with other children with disabilities, and thus, the need for careful research is critical. A better understanding of what type of social pragmatics programs really make a significant difference in helping the child with AS negotiate his or her social world, and the creation of prevention and treatment programs that are empirically determined would be critical contributions to the field.

References

Ammerman, R. T. (1997). Physical abuse and childhood disability: Risk factors and treatment factors. *Journal of Aggression, Maltreatment and Trauma, 1*(1), 207–225.

Barnhill, G. P. (2001). Social attributions and depression in adolescents with Asperger syndrome. *Focus on Autism & Other Developmental Disabilities, 16*(1), 46–54.

Batshaw, M. (Ed.) (1997). *Children with disabilities* (4th ed). Baltimore: Paul H. Brookes.

Bauer, S. (1999). Asperger syndrome. *Online Asperger Syndrome Information and Support,* http//www.udel.edu/bkirby/asperger/, 1–7.

Barnhill, G. (2001). What's new in AS research: A synthesis of research conducted by the Asperger Syndrome Project. *Interventions in Schools and Clinic, 36*(5), 300–305.

Belsky, J. (1993). Etiology of child maltreatment: A developmental-ecological analysis. *Psychological Bulletin, 14*(3), 413–434.

Bruhn, C. M. Young children with disabilities in the welfare system. Paper presented at the 7th International Family Violence Conference, Durham, NH, August 1, 2002.

Burger. F., & Lang, C. (1998). Diagnoses commonly missed in childhood: Long-term outcome and implications. *Psychiatric Clinics of North America, 21*(4), 927–940.

Clees, T., & Gast, D. (1994). Social Safety skills instruction for individuals with disabilities: A sequential model. *Education and Treatment of Children, 1*(2), 163–184.

Committee on Child Abuse and Neglect and Committee on Children with Disabilities. (2001). Assessment of maltreatment of children with disabilities. *American Academy of Pediatrics, 108*(2), 508–512.

Cook, B. G. (2001). A comparison of teachers' attitudes toward their included students with mild and severe disabilities. *Journal of Special Education, 34*(4), 203–214.

Crick, N. R., Casas, J. F., & Nelson, D. (2002). Toward a more comprehensive understanding of peer maltreatment: Studies of relational victimization. *Current Directions in Psychological Science, 11*(3), 98–101.

De Panfilis, D. (1998). Intervening with families when children are neglected. In HDubowitz (Ed.). *Neglected children: Research, practice and policy* (pp. 211–236). Thousand Oaks, CA: Sage.

Downie, S. (2001). Falling through the gap: Women with mild learning disabilities and self-harm. *Feminist Review, 68,* 177–181.

Finkelhor, D., & Asdigian, N. L. (1996). Risk factors for youth victimization: Beyond a lifestyle/routines activities theory approach. *Violence & Victims, 11*(1), 3–19.

Finkelhor, D., Mitchell, K., & Walak, J. (2000). *Online victimization: A report on the nation's youth.* National Center for Missing and Exploited Children. Office of Juvenile Justice and Delinquency Prevention. Washington, DC: U.S. Department of Justice.

Gazelle, H., & Ladd, G. W. (2002). Intervention for children victimized by peers. In *Preventing violence in relationships: Interventions across the lifespan,* Paul Schewe, (Ed.), Washington, DC: American Psychological Association, pp. 55–78.

Ghaziuddin, M., Weidmer, M., & Ghaziuddin, N. (1998). Comorbidity of Asperger Syndrome: A preliminary report. *Journal of Intellectual Disability Research, 42,* 279–283.

Gillberg, C., & Billstedt, E. (2000). Autism and Asperger syndrome: coexistence with other clinical disorders. *Acta Psychiatria Scandanavia, 102*(5), 321–30.

Grauerholz, L. (2000). An ecological approach to understanding sexual revictimization: Linking personal, interpersonal, and socio-cultural factors and processes. *Child Maltreatment*, 5, 5–17.

Greene, R. (1998). *The explosive child: A new approach for understanding and parenting easily frustrated, "chronically inflexible" children*. New York: Harper Collins.

Hazler, R. J., Miller, D. L., Carny, J. V., & Green, S. (2001). Adult recognition of school bullying situations. *Educational Research*, 43(2), 133–146.

Hollins, S., & Sinason, V. (2000). Psychotherapy, learning disabilities and trauma: New perspectives. *British Journal of Psychiatry, 176*, 32–36.

Huchet, C. G. (2001, Winter). Zero tolerance = zero thinking = zero sense: A school policy that places our kids at risk. *The Source*, A Publication of the Asperger Syndrome Coalition of the U.S., Inc. Jacksonville, Florida.

Klin, A., Volkmar, F., & Sparrow, S. (Eds.) (2000). *Asperger Syndrome*. New York: Guilford Press.

Lainhart, J. E. (1999). Psychiatric problems in individuals with autism, their parents and siblings. *International Review of Psychiatry, 11*(4), 287–292.

Lewis-Abney, K. (1993). Correlates of family functioning when a child has attention deficit disorder. *Issues in comprehensive Pediatric Nursing, 16*(3), 175–190.

Little, L. (2002a). Maternal discipline of children with Asperger Syndrome and nonverbal learning disorders. *American Journal of Maternal Child Nursing, 27*(6), 349–353.

Little, L. (2002b). Middle-class mothers' perceptions of peer and sibling victimization among children with Asperger's Syndrome and nonverbal learning disorders, *Issues in Comprehensive Pediatric Nursing, 25*, 43–57.

Little, L. (2002c). Stress and Coping of mothers and fathers of children with Asperger Syndrome and nonverbal learning disorder. *Journal of Pediatric Nursing. 26*(5), 1–6.

Little, L. (2002d). The ecology of victimization: Preventing negative health outcomes for children with Asperger's and their families. *The 2002 Hartman Child and Family Scholar Symposium*, New London, Connecticut, June 10, 2002.

Llewellyn, A., & Hogan, K. (2000). The use and abuse models of disability. *Disability and Society, 15*(1), 157–165.

Mansell, S., Sobsey, D., & Moskal, R. (1998). Clinical findings among sexually abused children with and without developmental disabilities. *Mental Retardation, 36*(1), 12–22.

Marini, Z., Fairbairn, L., & Zuber, R. (2001). Peer harassment in individuals with developmental disabilities: Towards the development of a multidimensional bullying identification model. *Developmental Disabilities Bulletin, 29*(2), 170–195.

Mazzucchelli, T. G. (2001). Feel safe: A pilot study of a protective behaviors programme for people with intellectual disability. *Journal of Intellectual and Developmental Disability, 26*(2), 115–126.

McCormick, L. (1995). Depression in mothers of children with Attention Deficit Hyperactivity Disorder. *Family Medicine, 27*, 176–179.

Mick, E., Santangelo, S., Wypij, D., & Biederman, J. (2000). Impact of maternal depression on ratings of comorbid depression in adolescents with Attention—Deficit/Hyperactivity Disorder. *Journal of the Academy of Child and Adolescent Psychiatry, 39*(3), 314–319.

Mitchell, L., & Buchele-Ash, A. (2000). Abuse and neglect of individuals with disabilities: Building protective supports through public policy. *Journal of Disability Policy Studies, 10*(2), 225–243.

Mullen, P. E., Martin, J. L., Anderson, J. C., Romans, S. E., & Herbison, G. P. (1996). The long-term impact of the physical, emotional, and sexual abuse of children: A community study. *Child Abuse and Neglect, 20*, 7–21.

National Center on Child Abuse and Neglect (NCANN). (1993). *A report on the maltreatment of children with disabilities* (DHHS Contract No. 105-89-1630). Washington, DC: Author.

National Clearinghouse on Child Abuse and Neglect Information (2001). *The risk and prevention of maltreatment of children with disabilities.* www.calib.com/nccanch/pubs/prevenres/focus.cfm.

Orelove, F. P., Hollahan, D. J., & Myles, K. T. (2000). Maltreatment of children with disabilities: Training needs for a collaborative response. *Child Abuse and Neglect, 24*(2), 185–194.

Raja, M., & Azzoni, A. (2001). Asperger Syndrome in the emergency psychiatric setting. *General Hospital Psychiatry, 23*(5), 285–293.

Rapin, I. (2002). The autistic-spectrum disorders. *New England Journal of Medicine, 357*(5), 302–3–3.

Reppucci, N. D., Britner P. A., & Woolard, J. A (1997). *Preventing child abuse and neglect through parent education.* Baltimore: Paul H. Brookes.

Richie, B. E. (1997, July). Gender, violence racism, and social marginalization: exploring intersecting oppressions. Presented at the 5th International Family Violence Research conference, Durham, NH.

Rourke, B. (1995). *Syndrome of nonverbal learning disabilities.* New York: Guilford Press.

Shirk, S., & Eltz, M. (1998). Multiple victimization in the process and outcome of child psychotherapy. In B. B. Rossman & M. Rosenburg (Eds.). *Multiple victimizations of children: Conceptual, developmental, research and treatment issues* (233–253). Binghamton, NY: Haworth.

Straus, M. A. (2000). *Beating the devil out of them: Corporal punishment in American families* (2nd ed.). Boston: Lexington.

Straus, M. A., & Stewart, J. H. (1999). Corporal punishment by American parents: national data on prevalence, chronicity, severity and duration, in relation to child and family characteristics. *Clinical Child and Family Psychology Review, 2*, 55–69.

Streek-Fischer, A., & van der Kolk, B. (2000). Down will come baby, cradle and all: Diagnostic and therapeutic implications of chronic trauma on child development. *Australian and New Zealand Journal of Psychiatry, 34*(6), 903–918.

Sullivan P., & Cork, P. (1998). Maltreatment prevention programs for children with disabilities: An evaluation model. *Developmental Disabilities Bulletin, 26*(1), 59–70.

Sullivan, P., & Knutson, J. (1998). The association between child maltreatment and disabilities in a hospital-based epidemiological study. *Child Abuse and Neglect, 22*(4), 271–288.

Sullivan, P. M., & Knutson, J. F. (2000). Maltreatment and disabilities: A population-based epidemiological study. *Child Abuse and Neglect, 24*(10), 1257–1273.

Tringo, D. (1970). The hierarchy of preference towards disability groups. *Journal of Special Education, 4*(3), 23–31.

Twemlow, S. W., Fonagy, P., & Sacco, F. (2001). An innovative psychodynamically influenced approach to reduce school violence. *Journal of the American Academy of Child and Adolescent Psychiatry, 40*(3), 377–379.

Weinberg, L. (1997). Problems in educating abused and neglected children with disabilities. *Child Abuse and Neglect, 21*(9), 889–905.

Chapter 6

Transition Support for Learners with Asperger Syndrome
Toward Successful Adulthood

Peter F. Gerhardt

Introduction

Although still a relatively new diagnostic entity (American Psychiatric Association, 1994), psychologists, social workers and educators are increasingly finding themselves asked to assess and/or intervene in the lives of adolescents and young adults with Asperger Syndrome (AS). From the educational preparation for life beyond the classroom to the development of strategies for promoting social access, to the management of possible co-morbid conditions such as depression, bi-polar disorder or obsessive-compulsive disorder (Martin, Patzer, Volkmar, 2000), the needs of persons with AS are complex, diverse and generally lifelong. Further, intervention options that address solely the identified skill deficits of the person with AS without addressing the social, educational and familial environments in which these deficits are most prominent may be, at best, only slightly effective. As such, an understanding of the adolescent with AS in terms of systems structure should prove helpful.

The Adolescent with Asperger Syndrome
in the Neurotypical World

Within the context of a society that values social competence, the communicative and social deficits presented by persons with AS represent a significant, life-long challenge to their ability to live, work, and participate in recreational activities as independently as possible (Harris & Handleman, 1997; Landa, 2000; McConaughy, Stowitschek, Salzberg & Peatross, 1989). However, during initial meetings, consultations, or job interviews many adults with AS may present as socially competent if a bit "quirky." There may be a tendency on the part of the clinician to perceive the disorder as "mild" (Tantam, 2000) and perhaps, to some extent, volitional in nature (resulting in AS often being referred to as a "hidden disability".) This, obviously, is not the case.

Such misperceptions are often based on either observations of relatively small samples of behavior (for example, a 20 minute doctor visit) or a misunderstanding regarding the nature of AS ("He can do it if only he would try harder.") Anecdotal reports (D. Vickers, personal communication, 2000; Sherry, 2000) along with some recent research (e.g., Hurlbutt & Chalmers, 2002) suggest that many individuals with AS experience significant levels of frustration with the inability of the "neurotypical (NT) world" to better understand and recognize how difficult life may be for them.

A sentiment often expressed at The Douglass Group, a support group for adults with AS that I founded a number of years ago was "If you NTs have all the skills, why don't you adapt for a while?" The perceived professional proclivity to focus solely on somehow "changing" the person with AS was often discussed as similar to expecting a person who is blind to see if only he or she would try harder. Given that, group members instead argued that while the primary focus of intervention should remain on the provision of skills to the learner with AS, the focus should be expanded to include comprehensive community education including individual specific environmental modifications. Thus, the area of intervention for the adolescent or young adult with AS would look something like Figure 1.

Another way of understanding this is to consider the difference between a disability and a handicap. A disability can be defined as permanent reduction in the function of a particular body part or structure. A handicap, on the other hand, is defined by the challenges that the disability presents to the individual's participation in desired, life-relevant activities. As such, the area of overlap in Figure 1 can be understood as representing the area where the disability that is AS no longer presents a significant handicap. Using this perspective, the learner with AS becomes

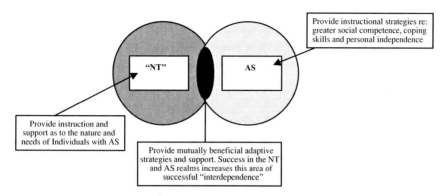

Figure 1. A Comprehensive Support System (Reprinted with permission from P.F. Gerhardt (2000). AS in adolescence and adulthood: Considerations for support and intervention. *New Jersey Psychologist, 50,* 26–28.)

one target of intervention among a variety of targets (e.g., teachers, classmates, co-workers, job requirements, physical environment, community knowledge, etc.) designed to lessen the extent to which AS, as a disability, results in a significant handicap. In this manner, more individualized and comprehensive systems of support and intervention may be developed (thereby increasing this area of overlap) and implemented across a number of domains including school, employment, self advocacy, and life skills including dating and appropriate sexual understanding and behavior.

The Issue of Social Competence

At the heart of the diagnosis of AS and, subsequently, any intervention is the issue of social competence (e.g., Tantam, 2002). But what do we mean by social competence? Gesten, et al. (1987) noted that social competence refers to a generalized "summary judgment of performance" (p. 27) across environments. Social skills, the authors contend, are subsequently best described as the discrete component skills of social competence, both verbal and nonverbal, that enable us to meet our needs and avoid unpleasant circumstances. Social competence involves the behavioral, cognitive and affective domains (Topper, Bremner & Holmes, 2002) and incorporates the fluent use of such diverse, yet discrete, skills as establishing and maintaining appropriate eye contact (micro-skills) and engaging in conversation and relationship building (macro-skills) (Gesten et al., 1987).

Further, social competence and its assessment are, to very large degree, context bound. As stated by Topper, Bremner and Holmes (2002),

"Everyone is socially competent in at least one situation and no one is socially competent in all." (p. 35). As such, any assessment of social competence for a learner with AS, on either a micro- or macro-level, needs to be recognized for what it is; a snapshot of abilities at a given time in a given environment. While this may help provide a direction for intervention, its utility in predicting success in different environments may be limited because of the differential social context of each new environment. As such, when the issue of social competence is discussed relative to persons with AS, there needs to remain an awareness of the temporal nature of competence as a function of both individual skill sets and the context in which the skills are utilized along with and how well this context either supports, inhibits or exceeds the skill sets.

In practical terms, this is of critical importance for the learner with AS at any major transition point (e.g., elementary school to middle school) but particularly as he or she begins the transition process out of high school. During the process, what was once a familiar, generally consistent, environment in the form of structured school day rapidly comes to an end. At that point, skills and abilities that may have been appropriate and functional during the school day may be ineffective and dysfunctional in future environments. Failure on the part of the individual's transition team to take this into account and to provide multiple opportunities to become socially, emotionally and physically comfortable, and establish some degree of competency, with the "transition to" environment offers reduced opportunity for the individual to succeed.

In the absence of fluent social competence however, addressing what may be referred to as social survival skills should be considered a necessary first step. Social survival skills are those base, minimum skills necessary for one to successfully navigate one's environment. In a way, they are sort of like the turn signals on a car in that knowing their use is truly necessary for safe vehicle navigation but hardly a sufficient condition for competing on the NASCAR circuit. For another example, we can examine the job interview process both from the point of view of social competence and social survival. Under ideal circumstances, a degree of social competence would be considered highly desirable during a job interview process (e.g., establish rapport, talk about last night's game, discuss alma maters, etc.). But in the absence of these skills, there are some social survival skills (i.e., establishing eye contact, smiling when greeting interviewer, avoidance of controversial discussion topics) that may be sufficient to highlight one's employability and allow one to gain access to employment. This relationship between survival skills and social competence is shown in Table 1.

Table 1. Toward Promoting Skills from Social Survival to Social Competence

	Emphasis Less Competence More Survival Necessary: Skills upon which independence may depend	Preferred: Skills that support independence but may not be critical	Emphasis Greater Competence Less Survival Marginal: Skills that, while valuable, may be negotiable
Riding mass transit	Wait until others get off before you get on	Whenever possible, chose a seat where you are not sitting next to someone	Whenever possible, put a row between you and other passengers
Lunch with coworkers	Eat neatly	Respond to interactions from co-workers	Initiate conversations with co-workers
Job interview	Eye contact	Ask informed questions about the employer	Comment on items in the office that may be relevant (e.g., is the person someone who likes to fish?)

Instructional strategies and packages for developing individual social skills and, to some extent, small areas of social competence have been reported in the literature (e.g., Baker, 2000; Barnhill, et al., 2002; Gray, 1995, Koegel & Koegel, 1995) What is less discussed is the importance of "individual outcome" as a critical variable in developing social skill repertoires. Social skills are generally recognized as functional in that their use results in either the receipt of positive outcomes or the avoidance of negative ones. That is, social skills are reinforced (strengthened) in individual repertoires by their naturally occurring consequences. A compliment offered to a colleague after a recent presentation may be reinforced by subsequently having greater access to the colleague and their work or by having them show interest in your work. For the learner with AS however, the desired reinforcement for offering the compliment may be an immediate and detailed 3 hours discussion on the topic. Anything other than that would be considered undesirable thereby reducing the likelihood of "compliment giving" becoming a fluent part of the individual's repertoire. As such, absent a clear understanding of what each individual might perceive as a potentially reinforcing outcome associated with the display of a particular social skill or set of skills, strategies to enhance individual social competence may be less than successful in producing lasting results.

The closest parallel in the behavioral literature would be the functional analysis of the conditions maintaining (usually problematic) behavior (e.g., Iwata, et al., 1982). In brief, functional analysis involves the manipu-lation of potential consequence conditions so that those conditions reliably determined to be maintaining the behavior may be further manipulated to effectively reduce the behavior in question. Of critical importance is that these identified conditions are highly individualized, potentially idiosyn-cratic and often complex in nature.

Similarly, those same descriptors (i.e., individualized, idiosyncratic, and complex) most likely apply to the conditions that support effective social behavior. Without a fairly comprehensive understanding of what an individual with AS hopes to get out of a friendship and in what con-text he or she expects that to occur, strategies to teach the development of friendships will only rarely be reinforced and, subsequently, generally ineffective.

For example, a number of years ago I worked with "Brian", an adult with AS, on the development of reciprocal conversation skills (i.e., em-pathic responding). At the time, the vast majority of his conversations revolved around his fascination with a particular mode of transportation. After a brief introduction to the skills and some roll play in reciprocal con-versation, Brian was able to consistently demonstrate the ability to par-ticipate well in conversations on topics not of his choosing. A few weeks later Brian and I were at the same social function and I noticed that every conversation he had that night, independent of the initial topic, quickly became focused on his interest in transportation. When I later asked him why he did not use the conversation skills that we had worked on, he re-sponded, "I know sometimes people find me boring and intrusive, but I find myself fascinating."

Brian, it seems, was not interested in making friends with someone who did not share his interests and so found little use for his newly ac-quired skills. If we had a better understanding of the function of friendship to Brian then the development of strategies that more effectively met his needs (e.g., how to more appropriately integrate his interest in transporta-tion into a conversation or how to better monitor his desire to talk about transportation) may have been possible. Again, the importance of under-standing the individual with AS within the context of the systems in which they live, work, and play appears critical if effective interventions are to be developed and implemented.

General Educational Considerations and the Post-21 Transition

Thomas Jefferson, in advocating for a system of public schools, wrote about the necessity of an educated populace if democracy was to work.

As a man of great foresight, he also argued that a system of public schools was necessary to ensure a self sufficient society—a society of people who could succeed on their own without government interference or support. Unfortunately, when it comes to learners with AS, minimal educational attention is paid to the development of self sufficiency beyond certain specific academic competencies (Klin & Volkmar, 2000) resulting in an adult cohort with significant needs and poor employment prospects (Gerhardt & Holmes, 1997). In particular, attention needs to be paid to the processes of transition to and from educational settings, to employment, and to competent adulthood in general including sex education, dating and self advocacy skills.

Secondary and Postsecondary Education

Klin and Volkmar (2000) argue that educational supports for learners with AS designed to foster social and communicative competence and promote appropriate behavior and emotional well being need to be developed and implemented in a thoughtful, consistent, and individualized manner. To that end, they list a number of specific recommendations for promoting self sufficiency as an educational outcome (Table 2).

Any educational plan for an adolescent with AS needs to address concerns relative to the post-21 world of possibly, college, and ultimately, work. Stephen Shore (2001), an adult with AS describes his educational journey through middle school and high school as increasingly less challenging until he entered college where he "never wanted to leave" (p. 77). He reports that the diversity of university life allowed him the opportunity to find individuals with similar interests and to pursue his own, particular interests in a more open and accommodating environment. Unfortunately, his case would appear to be something of an exception as despite a recent increase in the number of persons with disabilities attending college, retention and completion rates remain very low (Aune, 1991).

Among the reasons cited for this low rate of retention and completion are poor self advocacy skills, limited autonomy, inability to access needed supports (West, Barcus, Brooke, & Rayfield, 1995), and poor personal congruence between the person and their chosen program (Wilson, Getzel & Brown, 2000). Ideally, individual transition planning for success in college needs to begin far in advance of an individual's high school graduation year. When this not the case, there remain a number of transition strategies that when implemented during the later part of one's high school education, may help address these specific transition challenges. These include, but are not limited the following:

Table 2. Treatment and Intervention Guidelines

Goal area	Possible strategies
Problem solving	Specific as well as general strategies for problem solving need to be taught. These are often presented verbally but with significant behavioral role play involved.
Novel situations	Instruction on how to identify novel situations, assess such situations, and utilize a preplanned, well rehearsed strategy to address such situations. One such step might involve accessing a counselor's or other trusted individual's advice.
Social awareness	Instruction and support need to be made available across the day, not just during defined "social skills sessions".
Generalization	Programming needs to be in place to ensure that gains made in the classroom generalize to other, less structured situations.
Self-evaluation	Sometimes referred to as self monitoring, it involves training in the use of any number of social strategies coupled with the ability to determine which strategy might be best for which situation and, subsequently, assess how well the strategy worked and why.
Behavior	Instruction in identifying those situations that are most likely to result in anxiety, and the development of strategies to more effectively deal with them.
Adaptive skills	Skills explicitly intended to increase self sufficiency need to be incorporated into individual curriculums. Specific skills may include travel training, organization skills, budgeting, job maintenance skills, or dating skills as a function of individual needs, interests and desires.
Individual variables	For some individuals with AD, specific instruction may be derived from the result of neuropsychological assessments. Areas may include gross and fine motor, memory skills, visual-motor deficits, etc.

Source: Adapted from A. Klin, & F.R. Volkmar (2000). Assessment, treatment and intervention in adulthood. In A. Klin, F.R. Volkmar, & S.S. Sparrow (Eds.) *Asperger Syndrome* (pp. 340–366). New York: Guilford Press.

- Advance visits to campus to familiarize the individual with the general physical environment
- Coordination with other, non-university related agencies (i.e., governmental or local nonprofit) to access such services as case management, counseling, and housing support
- The scheduling of meetings with on-campus support staff to discuss expected challenges and potential needs
- The possibility of a "dry run" for campus orientation days or other, large social events (e.g., homecoming)
- The possibility of enrolling in one or two college courses prior to high school graduation

- A determination of the extent to which the individual in question is willing to discuss their disability with another in order to secure potential supports or accommodations (i.e., disclosure)
- The availability of some resource for peer information and training so that they may better understand the needs of the individual with AS

Employment Support and Training

One goal of any education is be able to be gainfully employed upon its completion. Unfortunately, for the vast majority of learners with disabilities, the goal of employment remains an elusive one (Sowers, McLean, Owens, 2002).

Because social competence is generally regarded as so integral to job success that it cannot be divorced from production competence (Hill, Wehman, Hill & Goodall, 1986; McConaughy, Stowitschek, Salzberg & Peatross, 1989) and many, if not most, of the difficulties experienced by adults with AS in the employment arena stem not from production-related challenges but rather social-related challenges. Given that, instruction and support for the adolescent with AS should include direct job-training experience, with emphasis on social skill development, in a supportive environment. Please note that this should be considered a critical component of secondary education even for those individuals for whom college is the immediate transition goal. "I know far too many adults with AS who have Ph.D.s and Masters Degrees and yet cannot get past the job interview because no one ever thought to teach them how." (Sherry Moyer, Personal Communication, 2000).

Sometimes referred to as job sampling, the provision of on-the-job or work study opportunities prior to graduation supports the development of skills such as job find strategies, interviewing, recognizing preferred and nonpreferred environmental conditions, and identifying potentially difficult social situations on the job. Direct instructional strategies relevant to these situations,—including role play, and possibly some self monitoring or related metacognitive strategies (e.g., Dixon, Moore, Hartnett, Howard & Petrie, 1995)—may then be more realistically developed and implemented on a case by case basis.

Beyond obtaining employment lies the issue of employment retention. As the myriad social skills necessary to succeed at a particular job may not be immediately identifiable, the availability of long-term (if intermittent) social support and social coaching may be necessary if employment tenure is to be a viable goal. This again highlights the importance of considering intervention strategies that are targeted beyond any individual skill deficits and address other, more systems oriented goals. In addition to identifying potential environmental modifications, the training of co-workers in the areas of: 1) the social and communicative needs of persons with AS; 2) promoting a socially inclusive environment, and 3) issues related to long-term employment support may help to provide an ongoing level of support to the worker with AS that might otherwise be unavailable.

Dating and Sex Education

Adolescents and adults with AS will generally require some degree of support and instruction in order to effectively navigate the world of independent living. Many of the activities that constitute life are straight-forward and, more or less, concrete. For example, there is little room for interpretation regarding how and when to pay bills, balance one's check-book, or which bus to ride to work. However, many other activities of daily living such as what do you do when you miss the bus or bounce check, how to avoid dangerous or uncomfortable situations are consid-erably more variable and complex, and perhaps none more so than the complexities associated with dating and sexuality

Direct instruction incorporating individual goals across multiple en-vironments is generally regarded as the intervention of choice for the vast majority of life skills for which one identifiable desired outcome (e.g., a balanced checkbook). But issues relating to dating and sexuality present a somewhat different challenge, in part because of their complexity, in part because of the potential risks that may or not be involved, and part because of professional avoidance of the topic having more to do with prevailing social norms than with the actual needs of the person in question (Tantam, 2000). While not all persons with AS are necessarily interested in dating or in the development of a physically intimate relationship for those who are, however, failure to address these issues should be considered inappropri-ate and potentially dangerous.

During another meeting of the Douglass Group, the question was raised as to whether men or women with AS labels experienced greater challenges in the areas of dating and personal sexuality. During the course of the discussion, the women discussed how dating was something that many were interested in but were not comfortable with. Unwanted touch-ing, feelings of discomfort and inadequacy, and even occurrences of date rape were discussed. The men in the group generally agreed except to add that when they make a mistake in this arena, perhaps something as sim-ple as saying the wrong thing at the wrong time, interpreting something incorrectly, or misunderstanding a woman's interest, they end up facing potential criminal charges.

Obviously, the issue is not a small one. As Jerry Newport (Newport & Newport, 2002), an adult with AS puts it, "The 'sexual explosion' hits us all. The realization that boys and girls are different and that there is a reason why, is a huge and often traumatic event for our people, with lifetime implications. It may be the most difficult issue for many families" (p. 11). It would seem, therefore, that instruction in that area personal sexuality needs to be addressed early, in a comprehensive manner, and inclusive of personal and family's values, the reasons and means to engage (or not engage) in consensual sex, and the reasons and means to avoid abuse and exploitation, if we are to meet individual needs.

Sex Education for neurotypical learners is not a "one shot" experience and neither should it be for learner's with AS. Comprehensive sex education should be viewed as an ongoing process beginning early in ones life. For example, the National Guidelines Task Force (1991) offers a list of relevant topics that should be addressed beginning as early as age 5 years. For children ages 5–8 years, the authors offer the correct names and functions of body parts, similarities and differences between boys and girls, family values and morals, and the avoidance and reporting of inappropriate sexual contact as potential areas of discussion and instruction.

For somewhat older learners, perhaps one of the most important considerations is the preparation of individual learners for the changes their bodies will experience during puberty. (National Information Center for Children and Youth with Disabilities, 1992) Females should fully understand the process of menstruation and appropriate menstrual care. Males might be instructed during this time regarding the importance of personal hygiene and provided information regarding nocturnal emissions. In addition, information regarding reproduction and pregnancy, abstinence, masturbation, STDs, and the importance of individual and family values in the decision making process may be made available at this time and should be presented in a manner that is accessible and understandable (National Guidelines Task Force, 1991). The Task Force authors further note that for older adolescents and young adults, the instructional path continues and includes such increasingly complex topics sexual health care, sex and communication, the impact of alcohol and drugs on sexuality and decision making, and personal responsibility.

Perhaps the most difficult and frightening issue for families is the issue of abuse and exploitation. According to Melberg Schwier & Hingsburger, (2000), this fear is often so palpable that parents and caregivers are often tempted to 1) deny the risk exists, 2) deny an individual's access to possible relationships, and/or, 3) deny an individual's right to be competent, involved adult. This third denial, the authors note, is potentially the most dangerous in that "keeping [your children] 'forever young' will keep them 'forever victimizable.'" (p. 133).

While open, direct and comprehensive instruction regarding the avoidance of abusive situations may not be sufficient to ensure complete protection, it would certainly appear to be a necessary condition. From differentiating between public and private behavior and between good touch and bad touch to the development of the decision-making skills and advocacy necessary to avoid most potentially dangerous situations, instructional goals and supports need to be individualized and functionally relevant. In addition, the development of a familial atmosphere that encourages the open discussion of these issues may be of significant benefit in preventing or minimizing the potential for abuse or exploitation. As Mary Newport (2002), Jerry's wife, co-author, and adult with AS puts it, "Once you open a dialog it should be life long process. If you wait until it seems absolutely necessary, it is probably a bit too late." (p. 49).

Dating skills, the precursor skills to consensual sexual acts, present a similar challenge as they involve complex decision trees that are primarily social in nature. From asking someone out, to meeting families, to holding hands, to more sophisticated levels of physical intimacy, dating is often acknowledged as presenting a challenging task to even the most socially sophisticated Neurotypical learner (e.g., Browne, 1997). A family situation that supports the easy and open discussion of these challenges may offer the best and most appropriate support resource available. In that way, issues can be discussed as they arise, and mutually agreeable solutions/supports developed in a relatively timely manner.

In summary, with regards to sexuality and dating, adolescents and adults with AS need to be provided with sufficient information and instruction to: 1) identify and avoid potentially dangerous or compromising situations that may occur as the result of social deficits (Klin & Volkmar, 2000); understand the responsibilities and processes of dating and physical intimacy; and 3) how to access help or additional information when needed.

Emotional Awareness and Self Advocacy

As social isolation accompanied by self esteem concerns are often reported by individuals with AS (Howlin, 1997; Myles & Southwick, 1999), particular attention should be paid to addressing these needs in adolescence and adulthood. Although, as noted by Klin and Volkmar (2000), "insight oriented psychotherapy is not usually helpful" (p. 361) for persons with AS, problem specific therapy (i.e., cognitive behavioral therapy) and generally structured counseling can be of some value. The therapeutic process, the authors note, can be helpful in alleviating individual concerns ranging from the challenges of day to day living to the complexities of interpersonal relationships.

Directly related to the concept of self esteem may be one's ability to effectively advocate on behalf of one's self for one's needs. In fact, it can be argued that self advocacy skills are perhaps the most important skills that can be provided to the special needs learner as part of the process of the transition to adulthood. Specific skills relative to the self advocacy process may include, but are not limited to: 1) awareness of individual needs, strengths, rights, responsibilities and accommodations; 2) awareness of individual acts of discrimination; 3) awareness of possible solutions to problems; 4) significant planning and coordination; 5) the desire to work hard on one's behalf, and; 6) perseverance (Gerhardt, 1999).

The ability to effectively advocate on one's own behalf can directly impact multiple aspects of one's life and is directly relevant to supporting an individually determined, positive quality-of-life (QOL). QOL, according to Shalock and Jensen (1986) constitues the goodness-of-fit between persons and their environment; and this goodness-of-fit can be understood as occuring along the complimentary paradigms of competence, choice, and control (Heal, Borthwick-Duffy & Saunders, 1996). In brief, we all require some degree of choice in our lives, some degree of control over our lives, and some opportunity to demonstrate competencies both across environments and time. Therefore, in providing services to individuals with AS, psychologists and other support personnel need to assess individual concerns not only from the point of view of normative society (i.e., the expected demands of the environment), but also from the goodness-of-fit between the person, his or her environment, and the desired QOL outcome.

Summary

Children with AS grow up and become adults with AS. With this transition to the world of adult interactions, demands, activities and privileges come multiple challenges. By understanding the needs, desires, abilities, and deficits of the individual with AS and their relationship to the demands of existing and desired environments, individualized and potentially effective systems of instruction and support can be developed. In that way, the once mainly academically competent student can begin the transition to become a more broadly competent adult.

ACKNOWLEDGMENTS: This chapter is based, in part, on a short article by the author originally published as P.F. Gerhardt (2000). AS in adolescence and adulthood: Considerations for support and intervention. *New Jersey Psychologist, 50*, 26–28. Permission, on the part of the New Jersey Psychological Association to reprint Figure 1 is both acknowledged and appreciated.

References

American Psychiatric Association (1994). *Diagnostic and statistical manual of mental disorders* (4th Ed.). Washington, D.C.: Author.

Aune, E. (1991). A transition model for postsecondary-bound students with learning disabilities. *Learning Disabilities Research and Practice, 6*, 177–187.

Baker, J. (2000). Social skills training for children with Asperger syndrome. New Jersey Psychologist. *50*, 21–25.

Barnhill, G.P., Cook, K.T., Tebbenkamp, K., & Myles, B.S. (2002). The effectiveness of social skills intervention targeting nonverbal communication for adolescents with Asperger Syndrome and related pervasive developmental delays. *Focus on Autism and Other Development Disorders, 17*, 112–118.

Browne, J. (1997). *Dating for Dummies: A Reference for the Rest of Us.* Foster City, CA: IDG Books Worldwide.

Dixon, R.S., Moore, D.W., Hartnett, N., Howard, R., & Petrie, K. (1995). Reducing inappropriate questioning behavior in an adolescent with autism. *Behaviour Change, 12*, 163–166.

Gerhardt, P.F. (2000). Aspergers syndrome in adolescence and adulthood: Considerations for support and intervention. *New Jersey Psychologist, 50*, 26–28.

Gerhardt, P.F. (1999). Self Advocacy. 10th Annual Supported Employment Symposium. Presented by the WVA Association for Persons in Supported Employment. May, 26, 1999. Flatwoods, WVA.

Gerhardt, P.F., & Holmes, D.L. (1997). Employment: Options and issues for adolescents and adults with autism. In D.J. Cohen, & F.R. Volkmar, (Eds.), *The handbook of autism and pervasive development disorders* (2nd Ed.) (pp. 650–664). New York: Wiley

Gesten, E.L., Weisberg, R.P., Amish, P.L., Smith, J.K. (1987). Social problem solving training: A skills based approach to prevention and treatment. In C.A. Maher & J.E. Zins (Eds.), *Pyschoeducational evaluations in schools: Methods and procedures for enhancing student competence* (pp. 197–210). New York: Pergamon.

Gray, C.A. (1995). Teaching children with autism to "read" social situations. In K.A. Quill (Ed.). *Teaching children with autism: Strategies to enhance communication and socialization* (pp. 219–242). New York: Delmar Publishers.

Harris, S.L., & Handleman, J.S. (1997). Helping children with autism enter the mainstream. In D.J. Cohen & F.R. Volkmar (Eds.), *Handbook of autism and pervasive developmental disorders* (2nd Ed.) (pp. 640–664). New York: Wiley.

Heal, L.W., Borthwick-Duffy, S.A., & Saunders, R.R. (1996). Assessment of quality of life. In J.W. Jacobson & J.A. Mulick, (Eds.), *Manual of diagnosis and professional practice in mental retardation* (pp. 199–209). Washington, D.C.: American Psychological Association.

Hill, J.W., Wehman, P., Hill, M., & Goodall, P. (1986). Differential reasons for job separation of previously employed persons with mental retardation. *Mental Retardation. 24*, 347–351.

Howlin, P. (1997). *Autism: Preparing for adulthood.* London: Routledge.

Hurlbutt, K., & Chalmers, L. (2002). Adults with autism speak out: Perceptions of their life experiences. *Focus on Autism and Other Developmental Disabilities, 17*, 103–111.

Iwata, B.A., Dorsey, M.F., Slifer, K.J., Bauman, K.E., & Richman, G.S. (1982). Toward a functional analysis of self injury. *Analysis and Intervention in Developmental Disabilities, 2,* 3–20.

Klin, A., & Volkmar, F.R. (2000). Assessment, treatment, and intervention in adulthood. In A. Klin, F.R. Volkmar, & S.S. Sparrow (Eds.). *Asperger Syndrome* (pp. 340–366). New York: Guilford Press.

Koegel, R.L., & Koegel, L.K. (Eds.). (1995). *Teaching children with autism: Strategies for initiating positive interactions and improving learning opportunities.* Baltimore: Paul H. Brookes.

Landa, R. (2000). Social language use in Aspergers Syndrome and high functioning autism. In A. Klin, F. Volkmar, & A. Sparrow (Eds.), Asperger Syndrome (pp. 125–158). New York: Guilford Press.

Martin, A., Patzer, D.K., & Volkmar, F.R. (2000). Psychopharmacological treatment of higher-functioning pervasive developmental disorders. In A. Klin, F. Volkmar, & A. Sparrow (Eds.), *Asperger Syndrome* (pp. 210–228). New York: Guilford Press

McConaughy, E.K., Stowitschek, J.J., Salzberg, C.L., & Peatross, D.K. (1989). Work supervisor's ratings of social behaviors related to employment success. *Rehabilitation Psychology, 34,* 3–15.

Melberg Schwier, K., & Hingsburger, D. (2000). *Sexuality: Your sons and daughters with intellectual disabilities.* Baltimore: Paul H. Brookes.

Myles, B.S., & Southwick, J. (1999). *Asperger Syndrome and rage: Practical solutions for a difficult moment.* Shawnee Mission, KS: Autism Asperger Publishing Company.

National Guidelines Task Force. (1991). *Guidelines for comprehensive sexuality education: Kindergarten-12th Grade.* New York: Sex Information and Educational Council of the U.S.

National Information Center for Children and Youth with Disabilities, (1992). *News Digest: Sexuality education for children and youth with disabilities.* Washington, D.C.: Author

Newport J., & Newport, M. (2002). *Autism-Asperger's and sexuality: Puberty and beyond.* Arlington, TX: Future Horizons.

Shalock, R.L., & Jensen, C.M. (1986). Assessing goodness-of-fit between persons and their environments. *Journal of the Association of Persons with Severe Handicaps, 11,* 103–109.

Sherry, L., (2000). A view from inside. In A. Klin, F. Volkmar, & A. Sparrow (Eds.), *Asperger Syndrome* (pp. 443–447). New York: Guilford Press

Shore, S. (2001). *Beyond the wall. Personal experiences with Autism and Asperger Syndrome.* Shawnee Mission, KS: Autism Asperger Publishing Company.

Sowers, J., McLean, D., & Owens, C. (2002). Self directed employment for people with developmental disabilities: Issues, characteristics and illustrations. *Journal of Disability Policy Studies, 13,* 96–103.

Topper, K., Bremner, W., & Holmes, E.A. (2000). Social competence: The social construction of the concept. In R. Bar-On & J.D.A. Parker (Eds.), *The handbook of emotional intelligence* (pp. 28–39). San Francisco: Jossey Bass.

Tantam, D. (2000). Adolescence and adulthood for individuals with Aspergers Syndrome. In A. Klin, F. Volkmar, & A.S.S. Sparrow (Eds.), *Aspergers Syndrome* (pp. 367–399). New York: Guilford Press.

West, M., Barcus, M., Brooke, V., & Rayfield, R.G. (1995), An exploratory analysis of self determination of person with disabilities. *Journal of Vocational Rehabilitation, 5,* 357–369.

Wilson, K.E., Getzel, E., & Brown, T. (2000). Enhancing the post-secondary campus climate for students with disabilities. *Journal of Vocational Rehabilitation, 14,* 37–50.

Chapter 7

Living with Asperger Syndrome
Real Issues, Practical Advice for Families and Helping Professionals

Sherry Moyer and Sheryl Breetz

This chapter has two purposes. The first is to explore several issues of importance for families with members diagnosed with Asperger Syndrome (AS). The practical advice contained within comes from the experience Sherry Moyer gained in parenting a child with AS and in helping others through her position as executive director of the Asperger Syndrome Coalition of the United States. The second purpose of this chapter is to use the success of a transitional youth advocacy project directed by Sheryl Breetz as a case study to encourage families and helping professionals in developing similar opportunities for youth with AS.

It was 1944 that Hans Asperger published his clinical observations describing a condition he referred to as autistic psychopathy. His ideas would go largely unrecognized in the scientific community until Lorna Wing (1981) published her landmark work and retitled the condition AS. She believed that renaming it would lessen the tendency for people to associate AS with mental illnesses like Schizophrenia.

More than another decade would pass until 1994 when AS was included in the American Psychiatric Association's *Diagnostic and Statistical Manual of Mental Disorders*, Fourth Edition (DSM-IV).

As is true with other recent disorders included or removed from the Diagnostic and Statistical Manual, the impetus for inclusion of AS was driven in part by parents and the early grass-roots AS family support groups that formed around the United States. There was nothing available for families needing support, and they were determined that they, as well as others, would not be alone in their search for appropriate information and services. A number of these individuals were also the founding members of the Asperger Coalition of the U.S., Inc. (ASC-U.S.) in 1997. The ASC-U.S. was conceived with the idea of becoming the national voice for advocacy issues as well as to support the numerous other regional and local groups that have been established over the last several years.

With this as background, we now examine issues of concern for individuals, families and professionals dealing with AS and its related disorders. Underlying each issue is a basic principle to be practiced by professionals, whether educators, mental health counselors, or medical personnel. That is, professionals need to empower families by nurturing the development of effective interpersonal and functional life skills in both the individual with AS and their family.

The Issue of Diagnosis

Almost everyone who has a member of his or her family diagnosed with AS has a diagnostic horror story to tell. Although there has been marked improvement in this area over the years, there is still a general lack of awareness that makes it difficult for professionals to consistently and accurately apply existing diagnostic criteria. What this means is that the individual in question is likely to have been given incorrect diagnoses such as Attention Deficit Hyperactivity Disorder (ADHD), Bipolar Disorder (BD), or Oppositional Defiant Disorder (ODD), which can lead to interventions that are often ineffective and possibly detrimental. Even when the young person has co-occurring disorders, we find families expressing relief when the principle issue (AS) has been identified. Once this has taken place, the process of educating all parties involved and creating appropriate supports for the individual will begin to prove more effective. This, in turn, will help to restore a sense of control and competency to the family as a whole.

Counseling and Family Support Issues

The issues surrounding counseling and family supports are complicated because the needs of the individual and family vary across time, and no two children with AS will present their characteristics in the same way.

For instance, there might be a period of time when a child with AS is in "crisis" which essentially means their emotions or behaviors are out of control. This may be triggered by an identifiable traumatizing event like a family move or change in schools. It may also be something more difficult to recognize such as the long-term effects of isolation that contributes to depression or severe anxiety.

During a "crisis" period, a team effort of professionals and the child's parents are critical to reestablishing a sense of normalcy within the environment. This is not a time for long drawn out discussions so much as it is a time to assess the immediate issues to be resolved and perform any "damage control" that may be necessary. Often it helps to have the family members simplify their routines and activities. This is because when they are in crisis mode, the person with AS is intellectually and emotionally overwhelmed and unable to act appropriately because of demands that are perceived to be either excessive or unreasonable. It is a wise idea to remember that preserving everyone's mental health is more preferable at that moment than adhering to the daily schedule. In other words, if the current pace of the environment is not conducive to recovery then change it!

One last point to note in this section is that for many young people and their families, just having the need for special services places an enormous stress on the family as a whole. It is a real challenge for families to assess the situation and then initiate and maintain the support services required for success in their daily schedule. Professionals can provide a great service for the youth with AS and their families by helping them develop the coping and adaptation skills needed to achieve a level of independence best suited to their abilities. It is important to remember that the presenting characteristics of AS can change with a person's age and developmental level. Professionals must help families stay informed and flexible to address varying needs as they arise.

Relationship Issues

Relationships are a major concern for individuals with AS. For a moment, imagine yourself plucked from everything that is familiar to you and dropped into a totally foreign culture. Body language, tone of voice, semantics, pragmatics, and facial expressions—everything you use to gauge the effectiveness of your efforts to communicate is lost to some degree, if not totally. Does the person next to you understand you? Will you successfully convey your needs and ideas? Will you understand the needs and ideas being conveyed to you? How will you know these things with any degree of certainty? You won't in all likelihood ever know for certain and that is the reality for people with AS throughout their lives.

Young people with AS experience these questions everyday of their lives, even with family members. They may feel anxiety because of the uncertainty surrounding their social interactions. Due to a deficit in their ability to generalize from one situation to the next, it may appear as though (s)he has not learned from previous experiences and has great difficulty making or keeping friends because of this. The truth is the young person may feel like every encounter is new and that they have no experience from which to draw when making decisions on how to proceed.

In order to encourage interpersonal relationships for their children, parents frequently become social translators, interpreting the outside world and its ways so that their children interact more comfortably with their environment. The concern about this scenario is that parents can tire of the constant need to translate and given the repetitive nature of the process can come to feel responsible for their child's failure to get along with others. It is truly heartbreaking for a parent to know that their child has few, if any, friends. Thus, it is important for professionals to recognize this and support parents accordingly.

As the child nears adolescence, relationship issues become more complex. Because of the naivety and social ineptness associated with AS, young people often find themselves in the position of being exploited or, at best, without a clue as to what may be unfolding around them. With humor and feeling, Stephen Shore, elsewhere in this book, writes about his encounters grappling with dating issues with young women who would have liked to be more than just platonic friends.

Knowing that these communication problems make the person with AS vulnerable to exploitation, families and helping professionals need to make a concerted effort beginning in early adolescence to teach the youth with AS to recognize appropriate and inappropriate sexual behaviors.

One of the more complex areas involving relationships concerns the reaction of siblings to the individual with AS. It is quite demanding for a sibling to have to learn to tolerate their brother or sister's idiosyncrasies. They live in the same house and cannot escape in the same way that the neighbor children or schoolmates can. While they may feel obligated to love and protect their brother or sister in public, they would like not to be frustrated or embarrassed as often is the case. Siblings should always be given an opportunity to have their own relationships independent of the young person with AS. It is extremely important to allow them to have a safe private place to express their feelings about how they are impacted by this disorder.

Professionals should remember that parents are also spouses and that spousal relationships must not be overlooked when interpreting the family's needs. Hopefully, there is a common philosophy between the spouses on how best to deal with their child with AS, but there is certainly ample opportunity for disagreement on the best course of action. Families often feel inundated with information and opinions so it requires tremendous effort from them to exhibit patience and dedication to each other while they sort out what is helpful to them. As families are faced with the need to find the balance between work, family and this disorder, parents can readily see where tensions might grow if things don't go smoothly! Professionals should encourage the concept of learning to manage the issues effectively so that the issues don't take control of their family's life.

School Placement and Educational Service Issues

Over the years, decisions regarding how and where young people with AS are to be educated and what services they should receive have become a hotbed for discussion. Tragic stories from the past and even today surface with tales of academic placement for students with AS in classrooms for the intellectually challenged or for severely emotionally disturbed students. Minimal experience with the AS population and a lack of special education resources cause some school systems to place students outside of mainstream classes in the name of providing more service, not necessarily the right service. It is an unfortunate unanticipated consequence that many young people with AS develop behavioral issues in the classroom when not provided with the proper accommodations to mediate their environment. There is, however, reason for hope with the advent of services being developed from a body of research and practical experiences.

For example, the Hunterdon County Educational Services Commission has developed a model program in Kingston, New Jersey. Using the program Academic Curriculum Cultivating Effective Social Skills (ACCESS), two teachers per classroom work with eight students to develop their academic and social skills. Tuition is the responsibility of the local school system.

Academics are individualized based on the student's ability level in each subject area. Each week the student and teacher contract on the academic and social skill goals that are the focus of efforts for that week. The

Hunterdon program has an allied helping professional staff that includes a full time speech pathologist, a part time occupational therapist, and a mental health counselor. In addition to its classroom academic program, the school uses field trips to help students navigate their community, foster special interests, and expand student's social interactions.

Transition to Adulthood

Our society is still struggling to build service bridges for young people in need as they legally pass from childhood to adulthood but remain emotionally and socially at a far different place and time. As Dr. Peter Gerhardt discusses elsewhere in this volume, the lack of awareness regarding AS is the single largest barrier to proper service delivery for youth in transition to adulthood. In addition, there is a lack of legislatively mandated services specific to the Asperger community. It becomes clear that the need to advocate for services for this group is vitally important. At a minimum, an advocacy agenda would contain legislation to protect the rights and needs of this population in a number of areas.

Medical Supports and Benefits

While some health care insurers recognize a diagnosis of Pervasive Developmental Disorder or Autism, fewer provide coverage for those diagnosed with AS. This is related to the lack of parity in mental health benefits for individuals in the United States. Depending on the coverage, some insurers cover services like social skills training while others do not, and ancillary services such as speech or occupational therapy are provided sporadically at best. AS should be included as a diagnosis eligible for treatment services in all health care plans.

Community-Based Services

While school-to-work transition programs are required through the Individuals with Disabilities Education Amendments of 1997 (IDEA), they are not fully funded or administered appropriately for students with AS. While aspects of adult life can be supported through the Americans With Disabilities Act, it too is neither comprehensive enough nor consistently able to satisfy the needs of the AS population. Legislation prescribing appropriate services as well as funding to develop community based support programs like those described later in this chapter is needed in order to foster healthy independent living skills.

Quality of Life

What does "quality of life" really mean? We are reminded of the comment Temple Grandin (Future Horizons conference, Boise, ID, 2001), a brilliant and highly visible adult with AS, has made on many occasions that she knows she will never derive the same satisfaction that her neurotypical peers might from things such as spouses or children so she has learned to find it in the activities she can accomplish on a more cognitive level. She takes great pride in her work with the cattle industry in addition to raising awareness for the Autism community. In essence, life satisfaction is an individually defined personal statement not a fulfillment of the expectations of others.

Independent Living Issues

A part of becoming an adult in our society is living independently from your parents. In the United States, most older adults with AS have had to carve out a life without benefit of appropriate medical or social service interventions. It is frequently the case that these individuals were thought of as "odd," "angry," or "difficult." It is quite possible they would have never been identified as having AS except for their children or grandchildren having been diagnosed in more recent years.

It is appropriate to point out that most adults with AS prefer to think of themselves as "differently abled" as opposed to disabled. They will tell you "We would be very successful in the neurotypical world with a few adjustments or modifications to our environment." A distinct challenge for the family members and professionals who reside in this "neurotypical world" would be to set aside their predisposition to "fix" what we deem to be out of the norm. This holds true for many disorders beside AS, but one difference with the AS population may be that many individuals with AS are cognitively capable of performing impressive intellectual tasks if given the opportunity. Practitioners in social service delivery programs would be advised to remember this sentiment when they are working with young people to establish goals for their independence as adults.

Long-Term Implications

AS is a life long developmental disability. As with other chronic conditions, youth with AS must establish themselves with some degree of comfort and stability in their environments. This is true of any young person;

however, when you include the daily challenges of constantly having to assess uncertain surroundings and consciously choose—what may or may not be the appropriate response—it becomes much more difficult to use your proverbial "auto pilot." Reactions and responses don't always arrive innately. It is real work!

Preparation for adulthood should begin as soon as the diagnosis is received. Fortunately, attention is now being given to developing social skills curriculums that can be taught on a daily basis in school or used in therapeutic settings with practice and support from home. It is wise for everyone to remember that realistic expectations for the child's development should be made clear, agreed to by everyone involved, and remain flexible as the child grows.

From a parent's perspective, there are long-term care and estate issues to consider. It is possible that their child will never achieve the level of independence of their neurotypical peers. Although there are millions of families that are responsible for their loved ones on a life long basis and are successful, this does not mean that the initial reaction to this revelation can't be a bit overwhelming as the implications are realized. Clearly, there is no shame in seeking help in coping with this reality.

As the individual with AS ages, family members will need to respond accordingly. Even when the child reaches a comparatively stable level of functional capacity as an adult, the family may still have to face the need to actively parent their children on some level. In the most positive of situations, it might be as simple as being the "safety net" or "sounding board" needed to check themselves as the individual with AS navigates life. It might mean retaining guardianship of their adult children and making most of the everyday decisions for them.

One last point to touch on for families with children of any age would be estate planning. Nobody likes to think about his or her mortality but the process for estate planning when a disabled child is involved is critically important. Consider the possibility that if the individual with AS is receiving Social Security Disability Income (SSDI) when the parents pass away that they might very well loose their SSDI because the earnings from the estate exceed federal income limits for the program. An attorney with expertise in estate planning should be consulted so that the family can ensure their child's financial security after their death.

Having been introduced to the concerns of the AS community, we next examine a successful advocacy effort for transition services. While this case study does not focus on an Asperger population, it offers a blueprint of activities that can be used to advocate for increased services for young adults with AS.

The Connecticut Advocacy Project

In 1998 the North Central Regional Mental Health Board (NCRMHB), a broad-based citizen review and voluntary advisory board, began an advocacy effort to build consensus on how to assist Connecticut's youth and young adults with serious mental health needs in their transition to adulthood. The NCRMHB consensus-building project was supported by a Community Action Grant from the Substance Abuse and Mental Health Services Administration (SAMHSA) of the U.S. Department of Health and Human Services.

The $150,000 federal grant focused on developing model transition services for youth and young adults, age 16–25, with serious emotional/behavioral disturbances and/or emerging mental illness. Serious Emotional Disturbance (SED) is a diagnosis commonly used in both the educational and children's mental health systems to describe a wide range of functional impairments in school, family, or community. Transition services refer to those services specifically designed to help a young person meet the challenges of adulthood, such as completing an education, gaining employment, living independently, and adjusting to community life.

The consensus-building project utilized the Knowledge Development and Application (KDA) Life Cycle concept described by SAMHSA as a framework for getting knowledge into practice (SAMHSA 1999 Meeting Presentation). The six steps defined in the life cycle are

1. Issue definition
2. Knowledge development
3. Synthesis of exemplary practice
4. Exchange of exemplary practice information
5. Preparing communities for exemplary practice
6. Adoption of exemplary practice

In addition, the project used Mattessich and Monsey's (1992) best practices for building collaboration, which recommended the following four steps in building collaboration.

1. Bring together multiple groups of people, identify problems and opportunities, discuss different views, and develop an expanded vision of the solution and strategies to be employed.
2. Bring the recommendations of these groups to key state agencies and planning groups, and identify processes to remove identified barriers, and organize the effort for implementation.

3. Develop a joint implementation work plan and build support for it.
4. Create visibility and support by presenting the proposed policy and practice to key groups.

Several activities employed in the consensus–building project illustrate how these suggested steps were implemented in building collaboration.

Bring Together Interested Individuals

The focus on services for youth and young adults originated because parents had observed enormous developmental losses for their children who developed a mental illness as they were entering adulthood. A committee consisting of parents, adults with mental illness, and providers was formed by NCRMHB to investigate this issue. Because such concerns were found to be widespread, the committee expanded statewide and became the steering committee of the consensus-building project. Membership on the steering committee was always open to any interested individuals.

Involve Key State Agencies and Advocacy and Planning Groups

The committee grew to include members of all of the state's five regional mental health boards, as well as members of other major advocacy groups concerned with mental health issues in both the child and adult systems. The committee gained credibility when the Deputy Commissioner of the Department of Mental Health and Addiction Services attended their meeting to hear concerns. Such demonstrations of support brought increasing confidence and belief in the group's mission and caused NCRMHB to apply for the SAMHSA grant. In addition, key decision makers in the state were interviewed so that the steering committee could understand their concerns, ideas, limits, and issues still needing resolution. Commissioners and other officials were interviewed in state agencies serving this special needs population. Legislators and department representatives were invited to attend the kick-off conference for the project.

Create Visibility

Immediately after the SAMHSA funding was received, NCRMHB sponsored a statewide conference to publicize the grant and the consensus-building project and provide a common baseline of knowledge about the issues involved. The powerful presentations of the individuals who themselves struggled with mental illness corroborated the presentations of the national experts, captured the attention of the invited media, and became the focus of a feature article in the state's major newspaper. The article also encouraged other families, consumers, and providers to join the consensus-building project. Presenters at the conference established a framework and knowledge base regarding the needs of this population, the issues they face, and promising practices for serving them.

Gather Knowledge from the Community, Data, and Research

Project staff gathered knowledge from the community. The consensus-building project included participants from all major constituency groups: consumers of state mental health services, parents, providers of mental health services, teachers, college professors, employment specialists, and advocates from both the child and adult mental health service systems. More than 500 individuals were involved in interviews, focus groups, or feedback surveys in an effort to describe the needs from various perspectives and the exemplary practice that would address those needs.

Key groups and individuals were targeted across the state. Individuals currently receiving adult mental health services were asked to look back over their experiences and describe what kind of services might have helped them when they were teens or young adults. Youth receiving services in the children's service system were interviewed about current needs. Parent groups were interviewed in cities and suburbs.

It was determined that knowledge from the community was consistent with the knowledge from national experts in the field. The local information was powerful, provided personal testimonials and was corroborated by information showing that the problems experienced in Connecticut were experienced nationally.

Staff reviewed the literature and collected state data that supported the need for transition services. Several programs cited in the literature as exemplary for this age group were contacted for information or were visited personally. NCRMHB later disseminated their findings from this effort to increase public awareness of both the problem and the most promising solutions.

Garner Support of Key Advocacy Groups and Other Initiatives

Project staff participated in thirteen statewide planning and advisory councils to call attention to the needs of youth in transition. As a result, several state government departments and non-profit advocacy groups prioritized transition services for youth with mental health problems as an urgent need in 2000.

In 1993 when NCRMHB began investigating the special issues of young adults with mental health needs, NCRMHB members had not yet heard of the term transition services. They were simply focused on improving services for young adults and enhancing their ability to experience normal life development. By the year 2000, as a result of the SAMHSA grant project, transition services were clearly accepted priorities, because a common understanding of need had emerged. What began with a parent's questioning had grown into a statewide focus.

Achievements of the Project

The consensus-building project culminated in the development of the Youth in Transition Program jointly funded for 3.2 million dollars by Connecticut's Department of Children and Families and the Department of Mental Health and Addiction Services that serves adults. The program was implemented at four sites in the state and incorporated the elements identified during the consensus-building project. Managed by the adult system, the program was created for up to 45 youth identified in the children's system with emotional problems or emerging mental illness who needed to transfer to the adult mental health system. This program provides clinical services, vocational and educational supports, and housing. Housing options have varied from scattered site apartments to clustered apartments in a single building to more congregate living arrangements.

The development of the Youth in Transition Program was a significant achievement. In a follow-up evaluation of the program by the five regional mental health boards in the state, three major successes were identified.

1. Many of the young adults showed significant achievements, including employment.
2. There was an increase in collaboration between the children's and the adult mental health systems.
3. There were increasing numbers of staff with expertise with this age group as a result of the program.

Applying Lessons from the Connecticut Project
to the AS Community

The project directed by NCRMHB was a comprehensive approach, which provides an example of the steps that other advocacy groups might take. Clearly, advocates for individuals with AS must find key appointed officials who will listen and respond to them and legislators willing to support funding for needed services. Private or public study grants can help support planning efforts similar to the SAMHSA grant. Other actions that should be taken include:

Establishing Statewide Committees to Ensure Transition Services

States should be encouraged to establish committees to guide transition service development. Membership on these committees must include consumer and family representation from various special needs groups, including individuals with AS.

Raising Societal Awareness

Individuals with AS are virtually invisible in today's society with many states having no services specifically available for this population. Parents and other family members must step forward and organize on behalf of their children if this situation is to change.

Engagement of Individuals with AS in Service Development

Historically, the population to be served has had little to say about the types of services they will receive. This is unfortunate. Clearly, individuals with AS must be included in developing and choosing their own services. If individuals with AS do not like the kind of services offered, they simply will not participate.

Involvement of Families

Relationships with families are very important and need to be considered in any services. There may be significant family members other than parents. Parents, young adults, and providers need to come to agreement on the role for parents of youth and young adults with special needs.

Specialized Services

Specialized services and best practices need to be implemented for this population. Services need to build upon individual strengths and address issues such as medical, behavioral, and cognitive needs. Advocates can be instrumental in getting best practices enacted and pressing for scientific knowledge to be put into practice.

Basic Life Supports

Advocacy needs to focus on the basic needs for adulthood, such as housing, transportation, and jobs to ensure an adequate quality of life. There is a growing understanding in the helping professions that treatment does not work as effectively if other needs are not being met simultaneously.

Conclusion

In the final analysis, what is the answer for the Asperger population? Here's what we know:

What Works?

The answer to this question lies predominantly in the global increase of awareness that has occurred over the last 10 years. Early identification and intervention is another key to success. Another factor is the improvement in tolerance levels in our society and an increased understanding that differences are not necessarily deficits. Family support groups and social skills training help to reduce the isolating effects of dealing with AS.

What Are the Barriers?

Even with the recent progress that has been made, awareness of AS and the needs of its population among medical and educational professionals and legislators responsible for funding needed services still impedes successful service delivery.

There are not enough diagnostic centers, which are staffed with knowledgeable teams of multi-disciplinary professionals who are able to provide assessments and recommendations for interventions, with opportunities for on-going services.

School systems are largely under-staffed, under-funded and under-educated to adequately provide for the needs of children and youth with AS.

As is true with many other medical conditions, individuals and families are frequently forced to battle insurance companies to obtain coverage for required services because the companies do not recognize AS as a life-long developmental disability requiring continued medical or therapeutic supervision.

Most teens and young adults are not prepared for the transition to adulthood. Services are needed that focus directly on improving vocations and independent living skills. Youth are also not conversant in the ramifications of disclosure, which could require that employers make appropriate accommodations that allow these bright young people to succeed if they are told in advance of the disability. Stories abound of well-educated adults with AS with 20 or 30 jobs in their relatively short careers.

Last but certainly not least is the very real barrier to success created by caregiver exhaustion. Parents who are tasked with fighting for every inch of ground their children gain in the community have very little left at the close of day to offer in the way of positive emotional support.

What Can We Do?

Beyond the issues that are discussed in this chapter, there is one requirement that stands out above all—Unity. A unified force of individuals and families coming together to address medical, educational and legislative concerns has been a key element of success in other advocacy movements.

A unified concept among medical professionals for diagnostics and effective treatment protocols that can be consistently applied would make great strides in alleviating the current frustration and confusion surrounding AS. Continued efforts to define and refine a unified definition of best practices in the educational field must be fostered through government funding and persistent pressure at the local level from families that are not willing to accept haphazard approaches to services for children and youth with AS. A unified commitment is needed to address all of these issues and improve the quality of life for children with AS and help them mature into successful adults.

References

Mattessich, P.W., & Monsey, B.R. (1992). *Collaboration: What Makes It Work*, Amherst H. Wilder Foundation, St. Paul, MN.

SAMHSA, (November 1, 1999). Community Action Grant Program Meeting. Washington, D.C., presentation by Neal B. Brown, Chief of Community Support Programs Branch, Division of Knowledge Development and Systems Change Center for Mental Health Services, Substance Abuse and Mental Health Services Administration.

Chapter 8

My Life with Asperger Syndrome

Stephen Shore

Q: Where does autism come from?

A: In many cases, autism first makes itself apparent from what I call the "Autism Bomb." What happens? I was hit with the Autism Bomb at eighteen months. A child is developing typically for about 18 to 24 months, and then something happens. There is loss of speech and tantrums. It's the environmental withdrawal. You see self-stimulatory activities such as children repeatedly spinning themselves or objects, and you see obsession on special interests; wonderful behaviors you've all grown to know and love.

Where exactly does autism come from? There are many different ideas. I think there's a strong hereditary component, which seems to get triggered by something else—maybe a vaccination, maybe sensitivities to diet, maybe something from the environment. I believe in the strong hereditary component because as I work with children on the spectrum, as I go to conferences, I see a lot of what my friend, Jerry Newport terms as "APHIDS", and that's an acronym for "Autistic Parents Heavily In Denial."

Editors' Note: Diagnosed with "Atypical Development with strong autistic tendencies" Stephen Shore was viewed as "too sick" to be treated on an outpatient basis and recommended for institutionalization. Nonverbal until four years of age, and with help from his parents, teachers, and others, Stephen Shore is now completing his doctoral degree in special education at Boston University with a focus on helping people on the autism spectrum develop their capacities to the fullest extent possible.

So I'm working with this child who's on the spectrum, and I look at his father, and well, maybe it takes one to know one, but I say, "Gee, Dad, I think you're autistic." He wasn't thrilled about hearing that piece of information. But then, later on, the stories come out. Guess who wouldn't eat solid food until he was seven years old? Guess who was diagnosed—well, not really diagnosed—but on his psychological report in 1954 it says "The kid can't be autistic; he's talking."

Well, now we know, we call that AS. The father's realization of his own placement on the on the spectrum helps him relate to his child. They often understand each other perfectly. However, sometimes the challenges of their both being on the autism spectrum cause serious misunderstandings.

Q: *Can you explain, exactly what is autism?*
A: The website of the Autism Society of America looks at autism as a complex developmental disability, starting within the first three years of life. Autism is neuro-biological in nature and not caused by poor parenting. The *Diagnostic Statistical Manual of Mental Disorders*, 4th edition, Revised (2000) (DSM-IV-TR) considers significant delays of social interaction; communication, repetitive motions and restricted interests as hallmarks of the autistic disorder.

Miller (Personal communication, June 10, 2001), who I've been doing some research with, says it's anything that interferes with the central nervous system getting the needed information from the environment. This seems like a fuzzy definition, but it's quite descriptive, too (Table 1).

ASA (2001)	A complex developmental disability that typically appears during the first three years of life. Autism results from a neurological disorder that affects the functioning of the brain
DSM IV-TR (2000)	Social interaction Communication Repetitive motions and restricted interests
Miller (Personal Communication)	Anything that interferes with the central nervous system getting the needed information from the environment.

Table 1. What is autism?

Q: *Please explain the sensory issues associated with Asperger Syndrome.*

A: Just about everyone on the autism spectrum I've met has some of their senses turned up too high, other senses are turned down too low, with much sensory information arriving as distorted and unreliable. This can make dealing with the environment in an interactive manner, especially when transitions are involved, very difficult.

Most people perform transitions in their heads subconsciously because their sensory receptors are fairly good. However, people with autism or Asperger Syndrome (AS) get a lot of distortion; a lot of static, which just encourages us to stick to the same old routines because it is always easier to do what you already know. I term these overwhelming type of sensory overloads and distortions as sensory violations.

Let's use the example of hearing birds in the morning when you wake up. There are a lot of them where I live. A common reason why people don't like to hear birds in the morning is because their chirping is bothersome and are woken you up when they'd rather sleep. Well, for me, hearing birds in the morning feels like their beaks scraping across my eardrum. It's sensory overload or violation. Fortunately, I have the verbal ability to express myself properly and explain these violations. Or I can modify the environment by closing the window. But what about the child in school who is sitting in a classroom and his eyes are actually so sensitive that he can see the fluorescent lights above him flicker?

So here he is sitting in a room like the one we are in today, but for a person with visual sensitivities—it's literally like sitting in a room with a strobe light. How can we expect the student to pay attention to his teacher, or do class work?

As a result, the student gets out of the chair to shut off the lights. The teacher says "YOU! Sit down!" This happens a few more times, and he gets sent to the principal's office and is going to have to stay after school for the rest of his life because he's been acting up; "out-of-seat behavior" once again. When is he going to learn? In this example, what I'm suggesting is that when we see behaviors like this, which we don't understand—challenging behaviors—they just might be caused by sensory overload issues.

Vision is just one of the five familiar outer senses of sight, touch, taste, smell and hearing. There are also the inner senses; one is the vestibular which helps us keep our balance. There is much evidence indicating vestibular problems with children on the Autism spectrum. Another inner sense is the proprioceptive; that has to do with the muscles and joints. That's what lets you pick up a glass of milk and drink it without shooting it over your shoulder because you lifted it up too fast, or keeps you from breaking the pencil in your grip when you're holding it while you're writing.

I was lucky and was born with a better than average vestibular sense. I enjoy riding my bicycle on the ice and snow, but there must be something going on with my proprioceptive sense. I remember talking to a colleague about my interest in autism, and she said to me, "Well, you know, I've been keeping my eye on you." I asked her what she meant by that and she went on to say, "I've been watching you for the past two and a half years. I knew something was going on with you, and now this explains it."

Being a person with significant experience in special education, she knew what she was talking about. So she said, "Well, kind of in the way you move. It looks like all the parts of your body are not connected to your brain right." What she did unknowingly was to give me wonderful description of how a person with autism or AS moves their body.

Q: What are the different diagnoses of the autism spectrum?
A: I took this diagram from Bryna Siegel's (1996) book, *The World of the Autistic Child* (see Figure 1). I love this diagram because I think it presents the DSM-IV-R information very well. However, I think it causes some confusion too. The Autistic Disorder in one place, then there is Asperger's Syndrome, followed by PDD-NOS. Then, a parent calls me up and says: "Gee, you know my child was just diagnosed. Thank God he or she is not Autistic. She's going to talk. Everything's going to be OK. By the way, what does 'NOS' mean?"

That's right. "Not Otherwise Specified," and I think that causes more confusion than anything else. We will be much better off if we look at Autism as a spectrum, ranging from severe to light (see Figure 2). At the severe end is where we see the classical Kanner's (1943) autism; those eleven children that Kanner wrote about in 1943. He was talking about, this is what most of society thinks about as people with autism; nonverbal, rocking, perhaps in the corner, maybe being self-abusive. Towards the middle we see moderate autism, PDD-NOS. Often children that get diagnosed here have more awareness of the environment, there may be more receptive language and maybe some limited expressive language. At the lighter end of the spectrum, we see high-functioning autism and AS. A lot of energy gets put into whether high-functioning autism and AS are the same, or whether they're different. Or

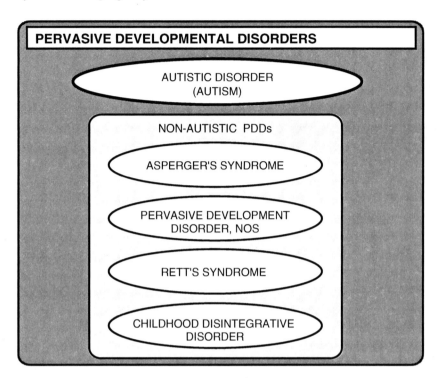

Figure 1. Autism compared with other disorders. (*Sources:* S. Shore (2001). *Beyond the wall: Personal Experiences with autism and Asperger Syndrome* Shawnee Mission, Autism Asperger Publishing Company, p. 146. Developed from B. Siegel (1996). *The World of the autistic child: Understanding and treating autistic spectrum disorders.* New York: Oxford University Press. p. 10. Reprinted with permission of the Oxford University Press.)

perhaps AS has nothing to do with autism at all. I like what I have heard Tony Attwood say at several presentations. He says that, "The difference between high-functioning autism and AS is the spelling (personal communication)."

Well, it might be a little bit of an oversimplification, but I think the idea is right, and that is, the issues still come from the same place. Whether you talk about autism or AS, there's still difficulty in socialization, communication, restricted interest, and one thing we need to get the people who wrote up the DSM-IV-TR, and other higher echelons, is the realization that there are sensory issues present throughout the autism spectrum. I was hoping that the revised version of the DSM-IV would have included sensory issues, but they didn't. Hopefully the DSM-V will.

Severe   **Moderate**   **Light**

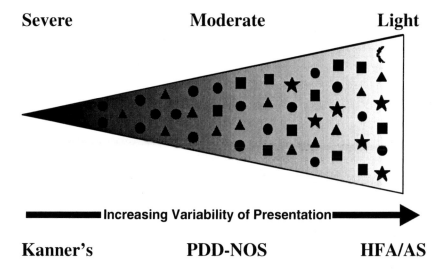

Kanner's   PDD-NOS   HFA/AS

Figure 2. The autism spectrum. (*Source*: D. Rosenn (1997). "Rosenn wedge." From Asperger: What we have learned in the '90s conference in Westboro, MA. Used with permission.)

Q: When should you tell a child they have Asperger Syndrome?
A: Often, clients will say, "I'm not sure that my son is aware that he has Asperger, that he has high-functioning autism, because we've never said it to him. And I'm not sure when it would be appropriate to say that. I'm sure he's aware that he's different, but I'm not sure." So the question is, "How old should a child be before being told that you've got AS, and this is what's making you different?"

I think it depends, with each child. There is no specific age, and the way you have to look at it is, first, their ability to handle the information, appropriately. This said, there are steps that you can take. You probably don't want to merely say, "You're a great son, and you also have AS, and that's it."

It may be better to start out by talking about differences. "You know, people have differences, and these are your collection of differences," and you leave it alone for a period of time.

Then you might come back later and talk a little bit more about it, and you might talk about the needs people have; some people need a cane to help them get around. Other people need an aide to help them get focused. And later on, you might say, "You know, there's a name for this collection of traits, and that name is AS."

But it really depends on the situation. Especially someone, like me, who likes everything ordered, I'd like to have a real nice, tight algorithm, just go step by step, this is what you do, and then, when you're all done, you have a disclosure. But people's emotions aren't that simple, so it's really more of a process, as opposed to at eight and a half years, and seven days, THAT'S when you tell them about AS.

Q: What really helped to you as a child?
A: At one and a half, the autism bomb hit with all of its ramifications. At two and a half, I got evaluated. It took my parents about a year to figure out where I should get evaluated. There were no conferences like this, no support groups, no books, except talking about how autism was some sort of childhood schizophrenia, and caused by bad parenting.

So I got evaluated, and got this wonderful diagnosis, of atypical development, strong autistic tendencies, and psychotic. And the professionals recommended that my parents send me away, to an institution. Why? Their reasoning was that my parents had a marriage to work on, two other children, and that the professionals would better take care of their child than my parents could. To which my parents said "NO—they're not going do that." And they argued with them and finally convinced the group—the team of professionals— to take me in a year. Maybe the doctors thought I would outgrow the autism.

The early intervention had to come from my mother, and again, I'm talking about a time when there weren't any resources; no support out there. So if you were to characterize what she did, in today's terms, we could call it a home-based early intervention program, emphasizing music, movement, sensory integration, imitation, and narration. And that may be why now I use music as I work with people on the autism spectrum and understand the importance of sensory integration.

My mother would try to get me to imitate her. That didn't work. Then she'd try imitating me, and when she did that, I became aware of her existence. And we see that, for example, in Barry Kaufman's (1979) book, *Son Rise*, where he and his wife sat on the bathroom floor, imitated and observed their son, Raun, for thirty-six hours until he became aware of them "Gee, you're there and part of my environment."

What my mother did with me, and later Barry Kaufman did with Raun, has very important educational implications; whether you're dealing with someone on the spectrum or not. That means you have to meet the student on their level. And if that requires you to get down on the floor, to stim or flap your hands with them, like I did with one kid to get him to know that I was part of his environment, then that's what you do. You don't do it all day, every day, but you do it long enough to let them know you're there, you're with them, and then you can pull them up into the direction that you need to take them.

What my mother did was to get inside my zone of attention. That's something we take for granted, and that has to do with environmental awareness. One of the key issues of autism, the autism spectrum, as described by Miller (Miller & Eller-Miller, 1989), is difficulty in body-to-environmental-awareness. Where do I end? Where does the environment begin? How aware am I of that environment, and also how fused am I with that environment? Do I realize that what's going on externally is really not part of me, or not?

Q: How do you teach someone with Asperger Syndrome to advocate for themselves?

A: I'm repeating the question. "How do you get someone to realize what their differences are from other people and use that knowledge to advocate for themselves?" Again, that has to do with awareness, of making a person with a difference aware that people have different strengths and challenges rather than "you seem to have problems with (whatever it might be)."

The challenge here is that you can have difficulty with something that most people don't have such as being in a room with fluorescent lights. So if there's a need to be in a room with fluorescent lights, you might want to go to the teacher or to your boss, and tell them "Well, gee, I've got sensitive eyes."

You might just leave it at that, too, because there's all different levels of disclosure. "I have sensitive eyes, and fluorescent lights bother me." Just leave it at that, instead of going whole hog, and saying "I've got Asperger Syndrome, and sensory sensitivities, and one of them, by the way, happens to be . . . "

That would be WAY too much information. As a matter of fact, if I decide to disclose my place on the autism spectrum when I talk about my book, I have a three-stage disclosure process. For example, my wife and I were at a faculty party. And the host introduces me, "This is Stephen Shore. He just wrote a book on the autism spectrum . . . "

A couple became quite interested. "Oh, you wrote a book on autism. That's great. What's it about?" My first answer will often be, "Oh, it's about autism . . . the autism spectrum or something like that." A lot of people say, "Oh, ok, that's very nice." And we'll talk about something else.

Or maybe they'll ask some more. That's stage two. "Well, what do you write about?"

And then I'll talk about visual aids in working with people on the autism spectrum, using music; issues adults face such as disclosure, education, and relationships. Sometimes I'll even say, that it's a text-based virtual reality tour of the autism spectrum.

And then, what I'll get from that is "Well, gee, that's great that you work with these children. You must have an incredible amount of patience." The third stage will be, if I feel that the person can handle and make use of the knowledge, I'll tell them, "I use the autobiographical form to . . ." and I will talk more about myself. Well, I was just about to enter stage two . . . and my wife says in a loud voice "Oh, he's autistic!"

Oh, gee whiz, thanks a lot! She beat me to the disclosure. However, that was quite an important step for her. When I first started getting interested in and working in the field of autism, she was afraid that my doing a presentation like this would cause all of you to run to the president of the college I was working at and I would lose my job. Now that's a little bit paranoid, but when you realize that she grew up in the People's Republic of China, during the Cultural Revolution, and people did lose their jobs for such things, then it becomes understandable.

Eventually, she began to realize of my ability to make a good contribution to the field, and became very supportive of my efforts. I remember that when I was writing my book, I hadn't found a publisher yet, and she kept nagging me, "When are you going to find a publisher? You got to hurry up and find a publisher! You have to finish your book before you graduate with your doctoral degree." Just like, you know, a Chinese/Jewish mother, all rolled into one. So needless to say, she was quite pleased when I did find a publisher, and now it's on to book number two.

My wife is very supportive of my traveling and doing these presentations, so the thinking has gone the other way, and I sometimes feel that if she's telling a few more people than I'd rather, about my relationship with the autism spectrum, but that's fine.

Q: *Can you give us some examples of the way people with Asperger Syndrome think?*

A: People with AS tend to think very literally. Here are some really good examples of how I used to think that might give you a good idea of how black and white things in our world are.

At age ten, oh, this letter "e"—, you drop the "e" before adding "ing", and there's a nice alphabet hanging on the wall above the blackboard, just like in most schoolrooms. And I just felt terrible for this "e"—how's this "e" going to feel? You drop it, it's going to get hurt, and I remember perseverating on that, for weeks to anybody who was in my vicinity. People didn't have a choice; they HAD to hear it.

Or a friend of mine who said he felt "like a pizza". "What do you mean—'feel like a pizza'?" And it wasn't until college that I realized, "Oh, he meant he felt like EATING a pizza." At this time, idioms usually go zinging past me but I am often able to "pull them back" for further examination before I say something ridiculous. But it takes some additional thinking, on my part, to figure out "Well, what's the meaning? How do I interpret this?"

Tell a child with AS to hold the door, please and this is what you get:

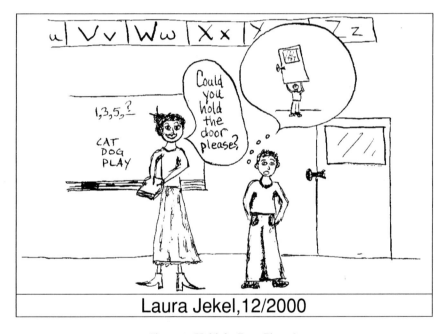

Figure 3. Hold the Door Please?

I remember when I was about nineteen, sitting in a restaurant with my parents, and they said to me, "You know, that girl over there, she's got her eye on you; she's giving you the eye." "WHAT DO YOU MEAN SHE'S GIVING ME THE EYE? I DON'T WANT HER EYE!" "You need two eyes; you see in stereo. She needs HER two eyes, that's gross and sickening anyway, and I won't take it." Idioms like that one got away.

Another time, I told a friend of mine that he gave an excellent presentation. He responded with "Oh, Steve, thank you very much, that was very sweet of you." I almost retorted with "What do you mean 'being sweet'? I didn't say it to be sweet, I said that you did a good job." Well anyway, I didn't say to him "Gee, I didn't say it to be sweet." I thought about it, but then I pulled it back, when I realized it probably wouldn't have been a good idea to start a debate with him about this, after he just finished a presentation and people wanted to talk with him.

Well, what if we translate that to middle school, and Robert, with "Asparagus" Syndrome... That's what I hear when I do a presentation at an elementary school, and soon I hear the children are talking: "Oh, oh, ASPARAGUS syndrome!" So Robert, with "Asparagus Syndrome," picked up a pen for Sally, and the teacher says "Gee, that was very nice of you Robert, you picked up her pen and put it on her desk, that's very sweet of you."

That is a very typical thing for a teacher to remark, and Robert says, "What do you mean? I wasn't doing it to be sweet! I was doing it because I thought it was a nice thing to do." And here you're seeing what's seemingly a challenging behavior; a person being rude, where it's really just a literal translation or interpretation of context.

Q: *What are some of the characteristics of behaviors that people with Asperger Syndrome can have when relating to others?*
A: Echolalia can be one such characteristic. That's the unintended imitation of sounds from the environment. I used to say I don't do that anymore, but while talking with a student in my office about a class I teach in special education, I suddenly notice that it's time to go to class. I log offline from America OnLine and the computer says "goodbye", to which I echo "goodbye." The student says: "OK, I'll go, I'll go. I'll see you in class." "No, no, you don't have to go, I'm just talking to my computer."

So, I guess it does happen. But what's more important to realize are the residuals of echolalia, and when I talk to other people on the spectrum about this, those who have written books, and present like I do, they have the same experiences. One has to do with imitation. "*I am telling you, I am veddy good at imitations.*" (said with the accent of an Indian guru) I love picking up accents, and imitating sounds that I hear in my environment, but the problem comes, is when it's unintended, and for example, my wife always knows who I'm talking to on the phone, because I sound like them.

I worked in a college where I had an African-American dean, and she had an African-American accent. And soon I'd start talking to her in this accent back at her. And she'd call me a brother, and I'd call her a brother; but actually I suppose I should have called her a sister. Then she'd call me a "homie," and I'd call her a "homie," and then I'd be horrified, thinking "Oh, I don't think I should be doing this; it's not really a good idea." Thoroughly embarrassed I stopped but never asked the dean if she knew I imitated her. The second residual is echopraxia, or unintended imitation of people's movements. Sometimes I feel like when I interact with the environment, I pick all these little bits and pieces of people's personalities, and they all get compressed and I use bits and pieces from these previous interactions here and there. I remember talking to someone about this. I guess it was the wrong person to talk to, because they said it sounded like I have a weakness of personality; that I didn't have a strong enough personality to create my own, because I absorb all sorts of other people's personalities.

Now the third one has to do with echoemotica, and that is taking on other people's emotion without realizing that it's not yours. We see this happening; we kind of know this happens anyway. We know that if we're in a bad mood, we get up on the wrong side of the bed on a particular day, we often think "Well, the children I'm going to work with are going to be off the wall. I just know it, and I'm not doing too well myself." Or, "My child is picking up something that's going on with me."

What happens is that we've fused onto another person's emotions, and haven't realized that emotion doesn't belong to us. And I know now, if I feel an emotion that's out of context with the environment, that I need to look around and say, for example, to my wife, "Gee, are you feeling upset today, or agitated?" Then she'll say, yes, she is. And once I'm able to do that, I can separate from this feeling of agitation. Now I still feel agitated for her, but also realize that it's not my emotion. So what I've done is cognitively built empathy in, you might say, a typical way. Then again, that has to be thought about, instead of occurring naturally.

Lack of eye contact is another real problem; what I say is "fake it, but don't break it." I'm not sure if people know when I'm looking between their eyes, or in their eyes, or at the bridge of their nose, or something like that. I think eye contact is a little bit overrated. I have a friend who does presentations like this, and he says, "I'll either give you eye contact, or I'll give you conversation, but you're not going to get both. Which one do you want?" (Jean Paul Bovee, personal communication, March 20, 2001).

Q: Can you teach a person with Asperger Syndrome social skills?
A: It is possible to approximate an intuitive sense of social interaction. The following analogy is from my good friend Philip Schwarz (Personal

communication, February 28, 2001). That's a lot of what we need to do. The social interaction skills of people not on the spectrum can be compared to a circle (Figure 4). It rolls very easily, you plop a nonspectrum person into a room with full of people and soon they are talking to other people.

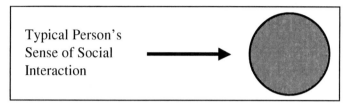

Typical Person's
Sense of Social
Interaction

Figure 4.

A person on the autism spectrum starts out with a square (Figure 5). You try to roll a square; it's got four bumps—and doesn't roll that well.

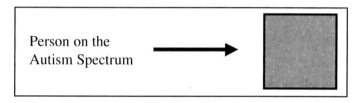

Person on the
Autism Spectrum

Figure 5.

We need to have algorithms (Figure 6). In other words, somebody needs to talk to us, about "this is what you do, this is how social interaction works."

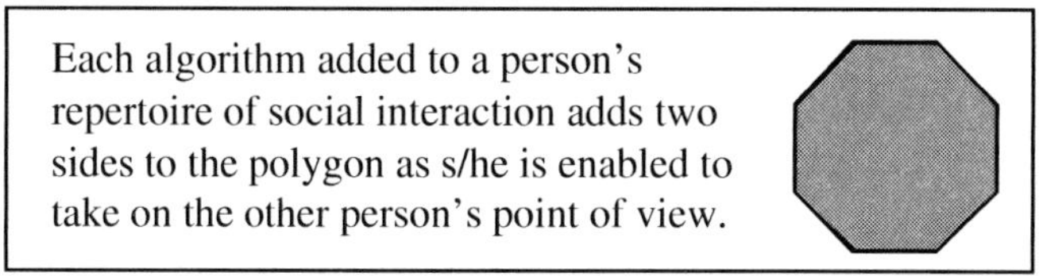

Each algorithm added to a person's repertoire of social interaction adds two sides to the polygon as s/he is enabled to take on the other person's point of view.

Figure 6.

These explanations can be done in the style of Gray & White Social Stories (2002). Social Stories are used to help teach people with AS the rules of social interaction. However, many people with AS often see through these stories, so it becomes more important to talk about social interaction more at an intellectual level, instead of making funny little stories about what you do when you're in a classroom and you have an answer to a teacher's question.

But the idea behind the social story is very good. We need to have algorithms to help guide us through social interaction (Figure 7). So when I told the person I was working with, with AS, "When people look at their watch, that means they're bored with what you're talking about. That way, you know that you need to talk about something else, or better yet, give them a chance to talk." Even though I told him that, ten minutes later, he's going on again about another subject for way too long.

I said, "Hey, George. I'm looking at my watch. What does this mean?" He thinks about it. Then I see the light go off over his head. He says "WELL, some watches have roman numerals, other watches have Arabic numerals, and there's a clock on the wall if you want to see what time it is."

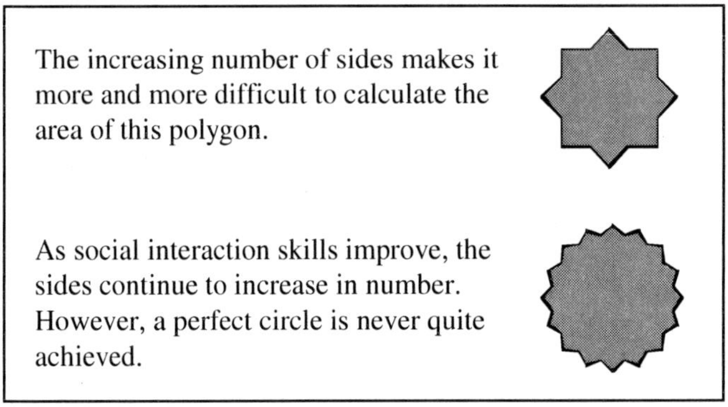

The increasing number of sides makes it more and more difficult to calculate the area of this polygon.

As social interaction skills improve, the sides continue to increase in number. However, a perfect circle is never quite achieved.

Figure 7.

Aiy, yahhhhh!! He didn't "get it." But the second time, the next week I saw him, he did have an understanding. And at the end of the session he said "You know, Steve, I noticed you didn't look at your watch. I didn't talk about anything too long. Everything I said was appropriate, wasn't it, Stephen? Everything was pertinent."

Well, that's another perseveration, but he got the idea. So as we keep doing this, we add sides to the polygon, but we never quite get to that perfect circle. However, we can get pretty close. And the shape would be rather bumpy if we used it for a wheel for a car (Figure 8).

"How does the sensitivity of AS relate to intuitiveness?" You mean about social interaction? "They may be more intuitive?" In some ways,

> Even though the polygon becomes ever more difficult to differentiate from a true circle, you still would get a bumpy ride if you used it as a wheel for your car.

Figure 8.

they can be. "Can they be more perceptive?" In some ways they can be. And it's almost always with people that they know well. That's going to be the subject of my third book. I see a lot of people with AS, and usually it's a son/mother combination, because it's usually boys who have it, and in this society, it's usually the mother that is deemed the caretaker.

What often happens is that the two of them get really tight, and close to each other, most likely from the fact that the mother has had to work harder with this child, either as part of the therapy, sometimes partly a therapist, teacher, and as an advocate. A lot more energy gets put into the whole situation—and that by itself often creates a tighter bond.

People on the spectrum can read another's body language, and their emotions, but it has to be someone that they're really close to. What seems to happen is that the son and the mother develop an atypically close, and some people consider pathological, relationship. This happened with my mother and I too. And it was almost as if we could read what the other person was thinking. That happens a lot.

And then somebody comes by and says "Well, if you just leave him alone and let him make his own mistakes, let him grow up, and leave him alone, let him make his own mistakes ... " Then the child with AS will fall apart. Because what has happened is that the mother has realized what accommodations need to be made.

And they see the accommodations, and often what happens is the child with AS will always check in with this person and now it's my wife, it used to be my mother. I talked about the issues of separation. That's also will be in that third book I mentioned earlier. This incredible closeness creates an additional challenge of separation. But it can't be done in a typical way. And it needs to be done with an understanding of AS. And what happens is, well, now my wife,—it used to be my mother and still can be if I'm with her—becomes sort of like a cultural mediator.

So, let's see what happens. A person with AS can't read a social situation, but I can the mother's, father's or other significant caretaker's face and body language. Based on this information and how that other person behaves, the person can take their cues on how to interact in the environment. So in that way, there could become an even greater sensitivity that can appear almost eerie.

Q: What about dealing with a child's special interests or passions?
A: What should I do about my child who perseverates on topics? Is it good or bad? Ah, perseverations. You gotta love them. Basically, the way I feel about perseveration is the school often looks at these certain behaviors, and says "These are bad. Let's push them away. After we push them away, then we can get to work" you might say.

What we need to do is to use the power of these perseverations, and in my case, it was bicycles. So let's get the child involved in a bicycle club, or if it's computers, can we get the child involved in a computer club? We can use that as a means to socialization as opposed to saying "None of this; you've done too much of this. You really need to get to work."

Sometimes though, these perseverations and special interests do become really excessive, and gets in the way of everything. Then we need to start thinking about saying things like "This is a good time to talk about dinosaurs, or this is not such a good time. Let's hold off until we get home or to an appropriate place." That's my take on perseveration.

At eight, I spent a lot of time cracking rocks. Smash open a small rock with a big rock, what do you get? Anybody ever do that? The rock splits open, and you see those little specks of mica and quartz, and it's a world unto itself, just like Temple Grandin (1995) mentions in her book *Thinking in Pictures* when she talks about spending hours passing sand through her fingers. Now this inside of a freshly broken rock is just a world into itself, and that grew into an interest in geology, and then geography, and various other special interests.

I remember, at about this time, a teacher saying that I'd never be able to do math, but somehow I learned enough math to teach physics at the college level. Another one said that I didn't know how to read. My parents said, "What are you talking about? He's reading the newspaper at home." So what they didn't do is pay attention to my special interests of astronomy and weather at that time.

What's a special interest? Tony Attwood (1998) says special interest is one of such great intensity that it interferes with daily function (1998). Does anybody know anybody with that type of situation?

SOME SPECIAL INTERESTS

airplanes	astronomy	bicycles	earthquakes
medicine	chemistry	mechanics	electricity
electronics	computers	hardware	tools
psychology	music	rocks	geology
geography	locks	cats	dinosaurs
watches	shiatsu	yoga	autism

Figure 9. Special interests. (*Sources*: A. Attwood (1998). *Asperger Syndrome*. London: Jassica Kingsley Publishers; S. Shore (2001). *Beyond the wall: Personal experiences with autism and Asperger Syndrome*. Shawnee Mission, KS: Autism Asperger Publishing Company)

Here are some of my special interests (Figure 9). They come and they go. Sometimes there is more than one of them is going on at once. But had the teacher realized, or taken notice, that I had a stack of astronomy books this high on my desk; well, maybe there's enough math and reading to be done in astronomy, at least at the elementary level.

Q: How about self-stimulating behaviors?

A: My concern is that a lot of parents and educators try to stop stims before they understand the purpose they serve. I tell them "You need to understand why your child is stimming, and then maybe you can substitute something for the behavior you find objectionable." The question is: "The child is hand flapping. Should I hand flap back at them and make them more aware of what they're doing?"

In a lot of cases, that will work. Sometimes they'll look at you and kind of give you a strange look, like you have two heads or something—"What are you doing?" Yeah, that can help make them aware of it. That's the idea of getting into their world and pulling them out. "Maybe we shouldn't be hand flapping right now." Or you flap at them, and say, "Here, here's something else to do with your hands. This might be a little bit better, at least while we're outside."

I have a lot to say about stimming. Well, what is it? First of all, everybody does it. It's just that most adults have figured out how to do it in a more socially acceptable manner. Like shaking your foot up and down, those are all socially acceptable stims. So, where does it come from? Either the brain is overstimulated, and you need the regularity of the behavior to calm yourself down, or the other way, perhaps you're bored out of your mind at a meeting; and that's how you keep yourself awake.

Trying to squash a stim is sort of like stepping on a waterbed. This part goes down, the other part goes up. So it's not something that should be stopped, we should look at the martial arts and if somebody throws you a punch, you deflect the punch. You don't stop it cold. It is the same with a stim. So let's try to find a more socially acceptable way to stim.

Instead of flapping the hands, maybe some sort of squishy ball could take that place. Instead of bouncing up and down, like this, all during class, and making the chair and the desk squeak and disturb the class, maybe we should try putting that child on a therapy ball, which has all sorts of sensory integration ramifications. But, just to summarize, the act of keeping one's balance can help cause the child to focus. Instead of sort of having to bounce on their chair, or slinking into their chair and falling out of their chair because they lose contact with the environment.

So stimming isn't necessarily such a bad thing. And also, getting the child to realize where it is appropriate to do certain stims. I know people that just sometimes really need to stim, and during those times, they can find an empty room, or maybe even go into a bathroom stall to spin around. Make sure you flush the toilet when you're done so at least it looks like you did something appropriate in there, and that's it.

Q: How do you help youth getting ready to leave the school systems and transition to adulthood?

A: At age nineteen or so, a youth graduates thinking about college and perhaps making more friends. There is a big paradigm shift that needs to be looked at in the transition from public school to the community and/or to college. Often I see students leaving the public schools, where they had an Individual Education Plan (IEP), but they're not quite sure what that document is. Now they're done with that, though they've graduated—"No more special education for me—I'm going to be just like everybody else." Which then creates a disaster as they reach the middle of the semester with poor grades and the student realizing, "Well, gee, maybe there was something to that IEP and special education after all." And then they face the challenge of finding and going to the office of student support.

This brings up the issue of disclosure–well, have we worked with the student about disclosure? Importantly, disclosing with themselves that they have AS or any disability, whatever they happen to have. They finally find the office of student support.

"Gee, Mr. Counselor, I have AS. Can you help me?" What's the first thing that comes out of the counselor's mouth? It's either going to be, "What's that?" or it's going to be "Show me the proof." Well perhaps the student's last diagnosis was done in middle school, and that's much longer than 2–3 year limit many colleges and universities have for considering a diagnosis as valid. Also, who's going to pay for the diagnosis?

So now it's the end of the semester, and the person with AS very well may have had a bad experience with seeking accommodations. That person shouldn't have had such an experience, and the public school hasn't done what it was supposed to do, and that is teach the person with AS—well, anybody—all the tools to lead productive and satisfying lives. And that includes self-advocacy. Most people self-advocate without thinking, people on the spectrum, well, we need to be taught, and as a matter of fact, I'm all for getting the child involved with the IEP as soon as it's given, and that could be in kindergarten, or it could be in fourth grade, or whenever it is. Get them involved in the process, and work towards actually having the student lead their own IEP meeting. That's the eventual goal. There's a whole lot more to say about that. Come to my class in special education and you'll hear more about it than you care to.

Q: *What about relationships with the opposite sex?*
A: Dating—that's a whole other issue. Fortunately I don't have to worry about it anymore because today is my twelfth wedding anniversary with my wife. When I started dating in college I remember asking people questions like, "How do you know when... how do you know when you've gone from acquaintance to significant other?"

I'd get all these weird kind of answers like, "Well, you just kind of know." So I'd wonder, "Well, is it like catching a fish?" Because I remember fishing with my uncle, and asking him that question, "Well, how do you know?" And he said, "Well, you'll know. The fish makes a big deal about it."

How DO you know? And I remember running into some, well... I could have run into a lot more trouble than I did. Someone like me, who doesn't process social interaction cues, for example, is told by a person of the opposite sex, "You know, gee, I like to give hugs. I like to give backrubs." And as someone always seeking deep pressure, I was all for it. And this woman even asked me if I'd like to sleep at her house one night. "Well, yeah, ok." Then I woke up the next morning. That was it.

Shortly, I noticed she was really frustrated. "Gee Steve, what do you want to do?" She said. THEN it occurred to me that "Oh, I think she wants to be my girlfriend." "No, I don't want to be your boyfriend. Besides you talk too loud. You're one of those people that you hold the phone out at arm's length when you talk to them." Talk about an aural overload violation!

And what has happened is, I guess I've been very lucky that the woman who became my wife had to use the cranial concussive therapy method . . . in order to let me know her intentions, and that's what my wife did. We had met as music students, with master's degrees in music, and started out with what I now call homework dates. We'd agree to meet in a certain place, do our homework, check each other's homework, split, and then eventually we started doing things together. She invited me to a Chinese New Year—she's Chinese—and I went to that and had a good time learning about another culture's ways and food.

I invited her to a few things, and later on, to a musical event at my parents' home. On the way there, she asked to stop in Plymouth to see the ocean. Well, ok, I like the ocean, too, so I agreed. So we walked to the end of a long pier and she gave me a big hug; that's good, speak through deep pressure, sensory integration. She then gave me a kiss, but by about that time I had realized "Oh, you could almost make a Gray & White (2002) social story about it. When a woman hugs you, they give you a tight hug and give you a kiss, it probably means they want to be your girlfriend. This is how you should respond . . . " So, I by the time my wife and I started dating, I had finally caught on.

There is much hope for people on the autism spectrum since an autism spectrum diagnosis is not a static diagnosis. For the most part, children diagnosed with an autism spectrum disorder will move towards the lighter portion of the autism spectrum. The challenge to all that work with this population is to bring them as far and as fast as possible to this lighter end of the spectrum. At this time we don't know all of the answers to working successfully with children on the autism spectrum, however, the following variables seem to have a large effect: appropriate early intervention, family support and love that accepts a person with autism as they are along with wanting to help them better interact with the environment, proper education, friends as well as teachers and other professionals that truly understand the child with autism.

References

Autism Society of America, *What is autism?* Website, accessed on January 13, 2001 at www.autism-society.org.

American Psychiatric Association. (2000). *Diagnostic and statistical manual of mental disorders of the American Psychiatric Association* (4th. ed., Text Revision). Washington, DC: Author.

Attwood, A. (1998). *Asperger Syndrome*. London: Jessica Kingsley Publishers.

Grandin, T. (1995). *Thinking in pictures: And other reports from my life with autism*. New York: Doubleday.

Gray, C., & White, A. (2002). *My social stories book*: London: Jessica Kingsley Publishers.

Kanner, L. (1943). Autistic disturbances of affective content. *Nervous Child, 2*, 217–50.

Kaufman, B. (1979). *Son-rise.* New York: Warner Books.

Miller, A., & Eller-Miller, E. (1989). *From ritual to repertoire: A cognitive-developmental systems approach with behavior-disordered children*. New York: Wiley-Interscience.

Rosenn, D. (1997). "Rosenn wedge." From Aspergers: What we have learned in the '90s conference in Westboro, MA.

Shore, S. (2001). *Beyond the wall: Personal Experiences with autism and Asperger Syndrome.* Shawnee Mission, KS: Autism Asperger Publishing Company. p. 146. Developed from Siegel, B. (1996). *The world of the autistic child: Understanding and treating autistic spectrum disorders*. New York: Oxford University Press. p. 10. Printed with permission from Oxford University Press.

Siegel, B. (1996). *The world of the autistic child: Understanding and treating autistic spectrum disorders*. New York: Oxford University Press.

About the Editors

Raymond W. DuCharme, Ph.D. is the founder and director of The Learning Clinic, Inc. (TLC), a private nonprofit education and treatment program for children and adolescents. TLC has provided day education and residential services since 1980. Dr. DuCharme has been a researcher and teacher, Adjunct Professor at The University of Connecticut and Assistant Professor at Brown University. He is a national consultant and author of numerous papers and articles on the subjects of treating and educating students with Autistic spectrum disorders and associated comorbid conditions.

Thomas P. Gullotta is Chief Executive Officer of Child and Family Agency of Southeastern Connecticut and is a member of the psychology and education departments at Eastern Connecticut State University. He is the senior author of the fourth edition of *The Adolescent Experience*; coeditor, with Martin Bloom, of *The Encyclopedia of Primary Prevention and Health Promotion*; and editor emeritus of the *Journal of Primary Prevention*. He is the senior book series editor for Issues in Children's and Families' Lives and holds editorial appointments on the *Journal of Early Adolescence*, the *Journal of Adolescent Research*, and the *Journal of Educational and Psychological Consultation*. He is on the Board of the Asperger Coalition of the United States. He has published extensively on adolescence and primary prevention. He was honored in 1999 by the Society for Community Research and Action, Division 27 of the American Psychological Association with its Distinguished Contributions to Practice in Community Psychology Award.

About the Contributors

Sheryl L. Breetz, M.A., is Executive Director of North Central Regional Mental Health Board in Connecticut. Board members include consumers, family members, and providers who work together to stimulate development of needed services. During 1998–99, she directed a federal Community Action Grant from the Substance Abuse and Mental Health Services Administration. The grant funded a statewide consensus-building project which culminated in development of state-funded services to help youth and young adults with serious mental health needs transition into adulthood.

Peter F. Gerhardt, Ed.D., is Executive Director of Nassau Suffolk Services for Autism which operates the Martin C. Barell School in Levittown, New York. The Martin C. Barell School provides educational services and supports to learners with autism, ages three to twenty-one, and their families. He is the author or co-author of articles and book chapters on the needs of adults with autism spectrum disorder, the school-to-work-transition process and analysis and intervention of problematic behavior. He has presented nationally and internationally on these topics. He currently serves on the Professional Advisory Boards of the Autism Society of America, MAAP Services, NJ COSAC, QSAC, and ASPEN. In addition, Dr. Gerhardt is the Chairperson of the Scientific Council of the Organization for Autism Research (OAR). Previously, he was a research assistant professor at the Rutgers University Graduate School of Applied and Professional Psychology with an appointment as the Director of the Division of Transition and Adult Services of the Douglass Developmental Disabilities Center. It was in this capacity the he cofounded the Douglass Group, a social skills and support service for adults with Asperger Disorder or High Functioning Autism. Dr. Gerhardt received his doctorate from the Rutgers University Graduate School of Education.

Liza Little, Psy.D., RNCS, is an associate professor of nursing and a clinical psychologist in the Department of Nursing at the University of New Hampshire. Her research interests include the impact of victimization on children and adults and the connections between the individual, and his or her family, and community. Her current research program focuses on understanding the victimization experiences of children on the autism spectrum, and the prevention of negative health outcomes for children with disabilities. She maintains a private practice in Durham, New Hampshire, where she consults to parents and children with learning and neurodevelopmental disabilities.

Kathleen A. McGrady, Psy.D., has been the Clinical Director of The Learning Clinic, Inc. (TLC) since 1994. TLC is a private nonprofit education and treatment program for children and adolescents. Dr. McGrady is a neuropsychologist and has been a researcher and author of numerous papers and presentations on assessment, diagnosis, and treatment of children and adolescents with autistic spectrum disorders, and the associated co-morbid conditions.

Jennifer C. Messina is a senior at Villanova University in Villanova, Pennsylvania, majoring in Human Services. Interested in after-school activities that promote the well-being of youth, she intends to work with young people after graduation prior to attending graduate school.

Sherry Moyer is the parent of a 14-year-old with Asperger Syndrome and the Executive Director of the Asperger Syndrome Coalition of the U.S., Inc. Before becoming the first Executive Director of the Coalition, Ms. Moyer served as President for one year. She has traveled throughout the United States, meeting with families and individuals to gain a better understanding of the needs of the Asperger population as a whole and help shape an appropriate national agenda.

Brenda Smith Myles, Ph.D., is an associate professor in the Department of Special Education at the University of Kansas, where she codirects a graduate program in Asperger Syndrome and autism. She has written numerous articles and books on Asperger Syndrome including *Asperger Syndrome and Difficult Moments: Practical Solutions for Tantrums, Rage, and Meltdowns* and *Asperger Syndrome and Adolescence: Practical Solutions for School Success*, the winner of the Autism Society of American's outstanding literary work. She is also the editor of *Intervention in School and Clinic*, the third largest journal in special education.

Jessica M. Ramos, B.A., Psychology, is a research assistant at Child and Family Agency of Southeastern Connecticut. She has served as a research assistant, editing, undertaking library research, and supporting the work of the editors Thomas P. Gullotta and Martin Bloom on the *Encyclopedia of Primary Prevention and Health Promotion*. She has also assisted in the editorial process for the *Asperger Syndrome: A Handbook for Professionals and Families*, and is involved in child observations and research for the Bingham Early Childhood Prosocial Behavior Curriculum.

Stephen Shore was diagnosed with "Atypical Development with strong autistic tendencies," nonverbal until four and recommended for institutionalization, Stephen Shore is now completing a special education doctorate at Boston University with a focus on helping people on the autism spectrum develop their capacities to the fullest extent possible. In addition to presenting and consulting internationally, Stephen serves as board president of the Asperger's Association of New England and as board member for several other autism spectrum related organizations.

Ann Wagner, Ph.D., is a clinical psychologist, is Chief, Autism/PDD Intervention Research Program at NIMH and is active in federal interagency autism-related efforts. Previously, she was codirector of an evaluation/treatment service for children with autism spectrum disorders and their families. She has extensive clinical experience as well as expertise in teaching and supervising clinicians in training.

Issues in Children's and Families' Lives

Series Editors:
Thomas P. Gullotta, *Child and Family Agency of Southeastern Connecticut, New London Connecticut;* **Herbert J. Walberg**, *University of Illinois at Chicago, Chicago Illinois;* **Roger P. Weissberg**, *University of Illinois at Chicago, Chicago, Illinois*

Series Mission

Using the collective resources of the Child and Family Agency of Southeastern Connecticut, one of the nation's leading family service agencies, and the University of Illinois at Chicago, one of the nation's outstanding universities, this series focuses attention on the pressing social and emotional problems facing young people and their families today.

Two publishing efforts are to be found within these volumes:

The first effort from the University of Illinois at Chicago Series on Children and Youth draws upon the multiple academic disciplines and the full range of human service professions to inform and stimulate policymakers and professionals that serve youth. The contributors use basic and applied research to uncover "the truth" and "the good" from such academic disciplines as psychology and sociology as well as such professions as education, medicine, nursing, and social work.

The second effort belongs to the Child and Family Hartman Scholars program. More than a decade in existence, this chosen group of scholars, practitioners, and advocates is formed yearly around a critical study area. This honored learning group analyzes, integrates, and critiques the clinical and research literature as it relates to the chosen theme and issues a volume that focuses on enhancing the physical, social, and emotional health of children and their families in relationship to that issue.

University Advisory Committee for
The University of Illinois at Chicago Series on
Children and Youth

National Advisory Committee for
The University of Illinois at Chicago Series on
Children and Youth

Index